Good Hair

Good Hair

The Essential Guide to Afro, Textured and Curly Hair

CHARLOTTE MENSAH

PENGUIN LIFE

AN IMPRINT OF

PENGUIN BOOKS

PENGUIN LIFE

UK | USA | Canada | Ireland | Australia
India | New Zealand | South Africa

Penguin Life is part of the Penguin Random House group of companies whose addresses can be found at global.penguinrandomhouse.com.

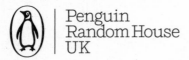

Penguin
Random House
UK

First published 2020

002

The information in this book has been compiled by way of general guidance in relation to the specific subjects addressed, but is not a substitute and not to be relied on for legal, accounting, tax or other professional advice on specific circumstances and in specific locations. So far as the author is aware the information given is correct and up to date as at 31 May 2020. Practice, laws and regulations all change, and the reader should obtain up to date professional advice on any such issues. The author and publishers disclaim, as far as the law allows, any liability arising directly or indirectly from the use, or misuse, of the information contained in this book.

Credit for in-text images: photo 1, Hair Growth Cycle: Shutterstock/Paper Teo; photo 2, Shape of the Hair: Shutterstock/Designua; photo 3, Skin Anatomy: Shutterstock/Designua; photo 4, Hair Anatomy: Shutterstock/Sakurra; photo 5, Hair Structure: Shutterstock/Paper Teo; photo 6, Hair Types: Shutterstock/cuppuccino; photo 7, hair: Charlotte Mensah, photographer: Kyoko Munakata, make-up: Neusa Neves; photo 8, hair: Charlotte Mensah, photographer: Kyoko Munakata, make-up: Neusa Neves; photo 9, hair: Charlotte Mensah, photographer: Krzysztof Grychnik, make-up: Nana Yaa Grant; photo 10, hair: Charlotte Mensah, photographer: Krzysztof Grychnik, make-up: Nana Yaa Grant; photo 11, hair: Charlotte Mensah, photographer: Sophie, make-up: Neusa Neves; photo 12, hair: Charlotte Mensah, photographer: Sophie, make-up: Neusa Neves; photo 13, hair: Charlotte Mensah, photographer: Krystoff Krychik, make-up: Sam Lascelle; photo 14, hair: Charlotte Mensah, photographer: Krystoff Krychik, make-up: Sam Lascelle.

Credit for plate section 1: © Charlotte Mensah + Lily Bertrand-Webb
Credit for plate section 2: Lily Bertrand-Webb

Set in 12.5/16 pt Dante MT Std
Typeset by Jouve (UK), Milton Keynes
Printed and bound in Great Britain by Clays Ltd, Elcograf S.p.A.

A CIP catalogue record for this book is available from the British Library

ISBN: 978-0-241-42352-3

www.greenpenguin.co.uk

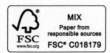

This book is dedicated to my father Seth Mensah
In loving memory of my mother Love Naa Densua Doodo
My grandmother Mary Owusua Thompson
My grandfather Michael Kofi Sefah (Dada)
This is my gift to you.

CONTENTS

FOREWORD

Charlotte Mensah is a *legendary* Black British hairdresser who combines the traditional techniques of her Ghanaian birthright with the Stonebridge Estate swagga of her Ladbroke Grove childhood. Her famous salon is also located right on the border between two worlds: close enough to Notting Hill to smell the Pilates but not so far from Kensal Rise that you can't hear a bell ring above a patty shop. From Willesden myself, I found Charlotte's in a moment of hair emergency. I think I found her by googling GREAT BLACK-BRITISH HAIRDRESSERS. Google is good for some things. And there she was, like an answer to a prayer. I'd been looking for someone like Charlotte a long time. As a kid, it was always my mum or auntie who did my braids, and I took their skills for granted, perhaps imagining they'd always be available for a seven-hour plaiting session, whenever I needed it, for all the rest of my days. But in college I learned that mums and aunties are not so easily replaced, and most British hairdressers were ill equipped to deal with my barnet. In the Toni & Guys of the period, for example, Black hair was treated solely as a difficulty: something to be blow-dried into submission. And I did that for a few years. Later, when I became determined not to submit my hair either to heat or chemicals, I set about the task of finding the one Black hairdresser who worked in whatever fancy salon, only to despair when, inevitably, they moved on elsewhere. But even when I could find that one Black hairdresser, I missed the atmosphere of those long-ago days sat on the floor between my auntie's legs, while lively conversations went on all around me, and everyone in the room knew what to do with my hair and did not stare at it as I freed it from a silk bonnet. It's this easy camaraderie and familiarity – sistahood – that you find at Charlotte's. She always makes you feel welcome. There's always tea and cake. You don't go to Charlotte to get your hair 'fixed' or 'corrected' – as if an Afro were a problem to be solved – you go to have your hair celebrated and cared for, oiled beautifully, braided perfectly, cut sublimely, styled to perfection.

In Charlotte's salon, everybody is treated equally, from the glamazon Nigerian girl who wants to look like Naomi, to the Jamaican pensioner in her Sunday best who wants her curls set, to the Polish woman with the little brown daughter who needs fresh canerows. The Notting Hill ladies of leisure have to wait just as long as the Kilburn gal who's come in on her lunch break. Waiting is an integral part of a Black salon, because Afro hair requires patience. In a Black salon there's always one woman kicking off because she thinks she's waited too long – you never want to be that woman. It's bad form. But even if you are, Charlotte won't get stressed, or raise her voice, or point out that good things come to those who wait. She will just bring you tea and nutmeg cake and carry on doing her meticulous magic to some other person's head until it's your turn. And if you just sit down and calm yourself and stop stressing you'll realize that waiting, in Charlotte's salon, is at least half of the fun. Pretty much every time I walk in there I come out with a short story. It's all-day characters, all-day chat, all-day drama, all-day philosophy and bare jokes, with Charlotte at the centre of it all, conducting twelve conversations simultaneously and only finishing about a quarter of her sentences before another thought strikes her. I could spend many, many hours there without getting bored – and I usually do, because that's how long Black hair takes.

Zadie Smith
March 2020

INTRODUCTION

Afro hair has come a long way since I started my career. In the 80s, I cut my teeth on the job, while working at the first Afro-Caribbean salon in the UK under the tutelage of Winston Isaacs, the godfather of British Afro hairdressing. At the time, the idea of natural hairstyles on the catwalk, or anti-discrimination laws to protect Afro hairstyles, was unthinkable; what's more, few hairdressers trained to care for our hair.

In 2018, after thirty years of service to the industry, I became the first Black woman to be inducted into the British Hairdressing Awards Hall of Fame. In the same year, the British media was talking about school expulsions for pupils with Black hairstyles and Lupita Nyong'o, a dark-skinned Black actress, was on the cover of glossy magazines, her natural, tightly coiled 4C hair reaching up to the heavens. Today, my list of clients includes trailblazing women like Chimamanda Ngozi Adichie, Zadie Smith, Janelle Monáe and Erykah Badu. I've flown the world over and have had women come from Berlin, Brasilia and Brooklyn alike to restore themselves at my West London salon, Hair Lounge. I've written features and been interviewed by *Vogue*, *Elle*, *Glamour*, *Stylist*, *The Pool*, *Grazia* and more. But here's the truth: I never intended to work in the beauty industry. As a teen, I had set my mind on working in finance. But sometimes your path simply doesn't run in a straight line.

Now a mother of two, I tell my children how funny it is to think about the things that you don't know when you're young. In hindsight, it's clear that a career in hairstyling was my true calling. As a child, my dada used to take me to his boardroom meetings, instilling in me the building blocks of business. And following the untimely passing of my mother, when I was thirteen years old, I took a keen interest in styling while caring for my baby sister's hair, and never really stopped. I went from apprentice to entrepreneur and business owner, recently launching my own range of hair products. The rest is history!

Today I'm ready to share both these stories and the wealth of knowledge I've gleaned during three decades spent caring for Afro, curly and textured hair. Looking after hundreds of women over the years has taught me a lot. About hair, of course: the scientific composition, the best way to tend to it and the different ways in which to present it. But my journey has also schooled me about business, family and what it takes to succeed: the losses, the gains and the life lessons that come with both.

In this book, I will tell you about my story and empower you to take ownership of your locks. Because it's not all about business. Hair feels almost spiritual to me, and I strongly believe that having your hair done is a form of therapy. It's a time to relax and to talk, if you need to, and to be, in a way, with family. Today I invite you to step into the chair and sit back so that I can tell you a little more about the art and science of Afro and curly hair. This book is a how-to guide, a history lesson and an intimate recollection of my life experiences, all rolled into one. It's a tool for getting to know, looking after and loving your hair. I hope whoever picks up this book – no matter their hair type! – finds answers to any questions they've ever had about caring for their hair, and hopefully a little bit of inspiration along the way.

Charlotte Mensah x

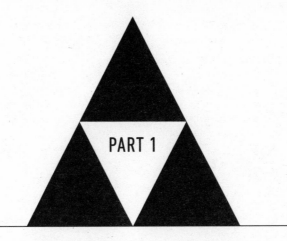

PART 1

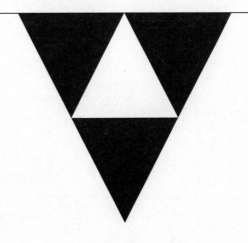

GOOD HAIR: AN EDUCATION

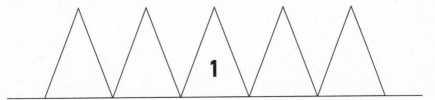

1

FROM MOTHERLAND TO MOTHER COUNTRY

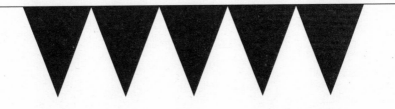

A BRIEF HISTORY OF AFRO HAIR

Before we start, let us go back to the beginning. The history of Afro hair begins in Africa, where the textures found on the continent are vast, from kinky to curly to straight, depending on the climate and the region. For at least 6,000 years – as far back as experts have managed to trace African combs[1] – the ways in which Black people style their hair have been a symbol of wealth and class, as well as profession and availability for marriage.

By all accounts, the rituals and habits surrounding Afro hair were as important in ancient times as they are today. Emma Dabiri, author of *Don't Touch My Hair*, writes that 'Yoruba braiding was already ancient in the 1600s'.[2] Over time, the diversity of styles has increased around the world. Many women in tribes throughout West Africa, especially Ghana and Nigeria, shave their heads after their husbands have passed away as a sign of respect. The Mende tribe of Sierra Leone took pride in women with hair that was long and thick because it signified their health, femininity and ability to procreate. According to African American art historian Sylvia Ardyn Boone, the Mende felt that 'a woman's hair must be clean, oiled and plaited. For the sake of elegance and sexual appeal, hair must be shaped into beautiful and complicated styles [. . .] Hair, to remain well-groomed, demands constant attention.'[3]

9

The Igbo and many other tribes carved combs made of wood for grooming, and these were made with long teeth in order to detangle the hair without pain. At the Hair Lounge, my salon on Portobello Road, I have many wooden combs from Ghana, proudly displayed behind a glass case. They're a symbol of my heritage and a reminder of our rich ancestral history. Hair dyes were made of clay, and adornments like beads and shells were used for ceremonies and rituals. Products were made of natural and everyday materials, such as plant extracts and animal fats, and palm oil or butter was used to moisturize the hair. Wealthy women in Senegal had their hair done every month in a style called the *gossi*, and they wove sturdy fibres, such as sisal, to lengthen their hair, applying butter and crushed charcoal before braiding.[4] In the mornings, women oiled their locks with petroleum and lamp black, a pigment made of carbon from the soot of burned fat or oil. Ayana Byrd and Lori Tharps, authors of *Hair Story: Untangling the Roots of Black Hair in America*, summarize it best when they say that hair for African communities acted as a gateway to the spirit world because it was the highest and most accessible part of the human body. In Ghana, I grew up hearing that hair was spiritual. You had to be careful what energies you were putting into it and trust the hands that were dealing with it.

Hairdressing on the continent was (and still is) a serious business as Afro hair lends itself to experimentation and sculpting practices that take time and artistry. Many styles still worn today, such as cornrowing, originated in Africa. Some styles – hair threading, for instance – are dying out. Both cornrowing and threading involve the etching of shapes and patterns into the scalp through the sectioning of hair, and these elaborate styles were used for important events or simply for aesthetics. The time women spent styling each other's hair was a time to share stories, laugh and come together as one, much like in the salon of today. Trust, love and companionship were exchanged in the doing of hair, which required long hours and patience. The Mende believed that the success of a hairstyle also had much to do with the energy of a space, which needed to be 'cleared of animosities and be full of good will and harmony'.[5] Byrd and Tharps state that the 'hairdresser was often considered the most trustworthy individual in society'.[6] Just like today, some styles took hours to complete, but unlike today, others could take several days, embodying a form of ritual. The authors elaborate to say that the Yoruba of Nigeria trained all women to braid hair but any young person who showed promise was made a 'master', responsible for the whole village's hair. When the 'master' died, she gave her tools to whoever came after her, during a special ceremony.

Hairstyling is an art – when you see a hairstylist at work, every single movement is precise and rapid. A good hairdo adds an element of glamour to what, for many people, can be a life of hardship.

Afro hair, in short, has always been sacred, a way to communicate with the divine, establish bonds between women and engage in creative (and healing) pursuits. It was not until explorers from

Europe came, between the fourteenth and sixteenth centuries, to trade (especially in human flesh) that the beauty and rich cultural significance of Afro hair was destroyed. Men, women and children were captured along the coast of West Africa, from Nigeria to Ghana to Sierra Leone, and sold as slaves. Many were forced to shave their heads, most likely for hygienic purposes, but the act served to swiftly remove identities and forms of self-expression, establishing a long and damaging history of control as well as negative attitudes towards our hair. Slave women, especially in the American South, worked in white households and were forced to keep their heads 'tidy' and 'neat' in accordance with European standards of beauty, which often meant straightened. Hair braiding then evolved from an art form to a means of practicality. Afro hair was described as 'woolly' by the dominant population and seen as ugly and generally inferior. Ayana Byrd and Lori Tharps write that enslaved men and women with dark skin and 'coarse' hair worked outside in the fields, while those with lighter skin and 'better' hair worked in the house, and these actions communicated ideas around 'good' hair and 'bad' hair, not to mention ideas around desirable and undesirable skin tones and features. As you will see throughout this book, these thoughts and feelings about Afro hair have continued to echo and shift throughout the ages and are still manifested, even today.

HAIRSTYLES THROUGH THE AGES

Afros and the Black Power Movement

The 1960s were a time of radical change, especially for Black hair in the United States and around the world, with the rise of the Afro. Instead of styling the hair using braiding or straightening techniques, hair was left as it is or in its natural state – to form a beautiful halo around the head, of various widths and heights. The style was revolutionary for many Black people who were taught that their hair should be straight and conform to European standards of beauty. It was both an aesthetic and psychological revolution. Suddenly, natural hair was released and celebrated, a symbol of a new kind of freedom and self-expression, with college students, activists and celebrities adopting it. The phrase 'black is beautiful' descended from the 'negritude' movement (a word coined by writer Aimé Césaire), which celebrated Blackness among francophone members of the Black diaspora. In turn, this inspired anti-apartheid activist Steve Biko, who was a proponent of the Black Consciousness Movement.

The bigger the Afro, the better. Afro Piks or combs were used to do just that, but could also be worn in the hair as decoration. The Pik was mostly a styling tool used to create volume. It was vertical in shape and resembled the ancient combs of Africa. It gained traction in tandem with the rise of political groups such as the Black Panthers, both in the United States and subsequently in Britain, who were making inroads into equal rights for Black people across employment, education and housing. Many people across generations and ethnicities were shocked by the style, for its defiance and openly textured look. The hairdo, for many, still looked unkempt. But the natural look didn't require as much of a fuss as straightening the hair, which was now seen by many as a disgrace to the race. The Afro, in turn, became about brotherhood and sisterhood within the Black community and spoke of solidarity. In the US, the Black Panthers used the style as a symbol of their liberation, along with the raised fist. The Afro spoke of a new consciousness and a reminder of our heritage and roots. No other style has been able to do that so powerfully, and many legendary icons rocked the look back in the day, such as Jimi Hendrix, the Jackson 5 and Angela Davis. According to Ayana Byrd and Lori Tharps, 'a New York hairdresser named Camello Casimir, better known as Frenchie, helped introduce naturally textured black hair to the mainstream after cutting South African singer Miriam Makeba's hair in a short 'fro for the January 1960 issue of *Look* magazine.'[7] Although the Afro began as a political statement in the 60s, it later became a popular style by the 70s. The style grew so much that chemical processes were put into place to make straight hair kinky, and Afro wigs were created for those wanting to hop on the trend. The Afro as a political or popular hairstyle would eventually vanish during the 80s and 90s, with other hair trends taking its place. Despite the lack of Afros seen today, the natural hair movement has superseded it, with certain entertainers and artists displaying their natural textures, such as Lupita Nyong'o and Chimamanda Ngozi Adichie.

Due to the delicate nature of Afro hair, there are a variety of combs and brushes to use, suited to the structure of our locks. In ancient times, some combs were created to decorate the hair while others were used for styling. In the past, combs were usually crafted with important symbols that could be 'distinguished by tribe and were often imbued with cultural and spiritual symbol-ism'.[8] For instance, historically, the Akan community (who have used decorative combs since at least the seventeenth century, although most collected combs are dated to the twentieth) were known to create a comb with seven teeth because of the numero-logical significance of the number – for example, seven days in a week, the time it took God to create all things, as mentioned in the Bible. The width between the teeth of the comb and the number of teeth also varied, depending on hair thickness and length. Some combs were made with animals at the base, or significant deities, depending on the region and the religion of the tribe. In general, these tools indicated wealth, class and status, and could be so big that they were primarily used as house decorations rather than for hair use. The British Museum has a comb measuring 31.5cm in height. Combs have also been known to be made as gifts, and men often gave them to women, both in Ghana and the Caribbean, as a symbol of their love and affection. Although the combs of today are no longer as aesthetically beautiful or as intricate as the historic combs of the past, they're necessary for detangling and styling.

A modern popular example of this symbolism is the tool designed by Anthony R. Romani in 1972, which featured a Black fist at the base to commemorate the American Black Power Move-ment. Of course, as well as their symbolic value, combs play a crucial and very practical role in maintaining healthy hair. Using the wrong type can lead to unpleasant results. (Head over to page 213 for more information on what combs and brushes to use.)

WEST AFRICAN MIGRATION TO BRITAIN

In 1962, the British Parliament passed the Commonwealth Immigrants Act. The purpose of this law was to restrict migration from Commonwealth countries, and it had a particularly big impact on West African and Caribbean immigration to the UK. The act was later amended in 1968, introducing further restrictions. At the time, Black people all over Britain and across the world were beginning to express themselves and fight for fair treatment and equal rights, especially after extensive colonial rule and wartime participation in both World Wars.

Once known as the Gold Coast because of the gold found by explorers, my own homeland, Ghana, became independent in 1957. On the back of European settlement came a history of West Africans migrating to Britain for new opportunities and a supposedly better way of life. Even those at the top of the social ladder were leaning towards the Western way of life: some of the most prominent African chiefs had sent their boys to England to get an education.[9] The start of the twentieth century saw many African students studying medicine or law and enrolling at the universities of London, Oxford, Cambridge and Liverpool. Many young West Africans coming to Britain were taught in missionary schools where the colonial outlook influenced their desire to explore new frontiers. But when they migrated, students had a hard time adjusting to the British way of life, encountering prejudice, alienation and racism, with many forming African Student Unions within and beyond their universities.

Growing up, the most visible example of this for me and my peers was Kwame Nkrumah, who was elected as Prime Minister of the Gold Coast in 1952. Originally born in the motherland, he studied in America before moving to London in 1945 with the hope of completing a PhD. He attended the London School of Economics for a term before returning to the Gold Coast in 1947 to participate in the country's burgeoning independence from British rule. His participation in the Black community in the United States continued here in the UK, and most of his time was spent attending meetings focused on the state of Africa after European colonization. Nkrumah attended the 5th Pan-African Congress in Manchester in 1945, which is 'now seen as one of the significant events leading to the independence of many African countries, and other attendees included Jomo Kenyatta',[10] the first person in Kenya to take up the role of President, and a fellow LSE graduate.

The end of the Second World War became a harbinger for radical change, both politically and culturally. It was during this transformative era that the Mensah family decided to make their way from Ghana to the United Kingdom – from the motherland to mother country.

Seth and Love: my parents' migration story

My very own story begins on the 22nd of May 1970, at St Mary's Hospital in London. My parents, Seth and Love Mensah, shared a single room in Maida Vale, a West London neighbourhood too quiet for a baby like me. Mum and Dad were trying to make ends meet, having arrived from Ghana to Britain in 1968. Dad had been a saxophone player in the motherland for a band called the Ramblers, but his parents couldn't see a future for him as a musician, and they put pressure on him to move to the UK to look for 'proper' work. Mum joined him four months later, and soon after that I arrived, their first child born abroad. My other siblings remained in Ghana under the care of my grandma and grandpa. Dad took a job at the Grosvenor House Hotel, washing dishes, when he realized how difficult it would be to find work. The types of positions offered to African immigrants at the time were limited and, in those days, Black people weren't allowed to stay in the hotel and were mostly hired as chambermaids or dishwashers.

Dad had never washed a plate in his life. He had to learn quickly, as a lot was expected of him. Oftentimes, he worked double shifts – seventeen hours a day. Meanwhile, Mum stayed home to look after me, but she would soon need to find work too. The stress of paying bills, looking after a young child and the cultural obligation of sending money back home to the rest of the family took its toll. Mum was advised by friends and family to send me back to the motherland for proper care and so, at three months old, I arrived in Ghana in a Moses basket.

Word of the child who had just come from England spread quickly across the community, and I soon became the talk of the town. I lived with Grandma and Grandpa (whom I called Dada and Mama) on a compound full of other family members. There were close to forty of us, coming and going, including aunties and uncles, cousins and siblings. Dada was the director of Tata Brewery and was driven to work in a Mercedes. I remember him dressed in his *ntoma*, something kings and chiefs wore – a kind of cloth he threw over his shoulder with shorts underneath. Dada, from the moment I arrived in my basket, treated me as very special. I would even go as far as to say that he spoiled me. Not only could I eat on my own during mealtimes – not having to share the large pot of stew, much to the annoyance of my cousins and siblings – but he often took me to his boardroom meetings, from when I was as young as five years old! I remember entering a room full of leather chairs, with a large table, air conditioning and ceiling fans. I remember men in suits, carrying briefcases filled to the brim with dollar bills. After work, Dada often came back to the compound with goodies: biscuits, or a nice fried egg sandwich I loved, on buttered toast or tea bread (a popular Ghanaian sandwich, like a McMuffin but nicer). I often think that, along with Mama's grafting, those early experiences with Dada instilled in me the building blocks of entrepreneurship and business. People were constantly buzzing around the compound and there were plenty of kids my age to play with. I often took on roles of leadership, gathering my siblings and cousins around me to read to them, as I was the eldest by a year or two. I loved sitting the kids in a line and bossing them about. I wanted to be a teacher, or a mentor to them, but they mostly listened to me because they knew where I stood with Dada, who gave me treats that I could use to influence (bribe) them.

While Dada travelled and attended lavish events, Mama was a deaconess and she liked to be home looking after family, working or worshipping at church, which was a big thing in our house. Although they were both Christian, they belonged to different denominations, so sometimes I'd go with Dada to his church with all the burning incense and the congregation dressed in white, and other times I'd go to church with Mama and participate in all the traditional clapping and singing. Mama was a Wonder Woman: a deacon at the church and the head of several groups for women. Mama, a prayer warrior, found time to wake at the crack of dawn to spread the word of God. She walked and preached the gospel from the distance of, say, Notting Hill to Brixton, but she returned home just in time to wake us up in the mornings to get ready for school. It's not an exaggeration when I say that she was good at everything, a bit of a local

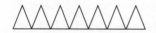

It's not an exaggeration when I say that Mama was good at everything, a bit of a local celebrity, well loved and respected. The type of woman who went above and beyond for her children and grandchildren, sewing our clothes, doing our hair, and managing the goings-on of the estate.

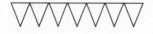

celebrity, well loved and respected. The type of woman who went above and beyond for her children and grandchildren, sewing our clothes, doing our hair, and managing the goings-on of the estate. Everyone knew her in the area for her freshly baked bread, which her grandchildren sold on their heads. The locals stopped us on the streets as we rushed like ants to sell the loaves quicker than anyone else. When we returned to the house, Mama gave us a commission for a job well done.

My mum, Love, was the eldest daughter of eight and she became the most precious child because she now lived in England. Mama wrote to her often by telegraph or sat with a tape recorder on a Sunday, after church, relaying messages on cassette about everything that had happened over the previous month with her children. Mum, in turn, would send suitcases full of provisions: biscuits, clothes and Avon products for Grandma and her sisters. The environment I grew up in was lively and full of activity, with Mama and her daughters cooking for their families in front of a coal pot. There were so many mouths to feed, they often fried up hundreds of fish or made big pots of stew to last three days. We all had to share the stew from a big bowl, and whenever one of the kids took too much meat, the rest of us would be angry. So if you were a slow eater, the greedy would eat everything and leave you well behind! We had a massive garden at the end of the compound where we grew our own produce, including yams and plantain, and reared chickens on the land. A mango tree grew too, and I remember the days when the fruit became ripe – and the fighting that commenced between us kids, as soon as the first fruit dropped.

From the age of five, I went to Harrow International, a mixed-gender primary school which was founded by an English woman involved in charity work. Mama and Dada had high expectations of me, and I was on track to attend the prestigious Achimota secondary school, home to some of Ghana's greatest minds. Students were very competitive about their grades and wanted to excel, and the teachers were focused on student achievement. Every day, school began with a prayer, and we often sang a lot too.

We had inspections every Monday morning, with the teachers making sure our socks were white and neat, our shoes black and smart, and our uniforms tidy. The headmaster could be very strict but at the same time fair. He wanted us all to succeed and he would push us to do so. In those days, there was a lot of physical discipline, such as caning, where you had to stoop down on your knees. Or sometimes you'd have to hold your ears out with your hands for an hour, and your ears and arms would be burning like fire. Our fingernails were examined for cleanliness and all students, boys and girls alike, had to have what we now call TWAs (Teeny Weeny Afros). Haircare for children was quite basic in those days, with Mama buying a tub of Dax (petroleum jelly in a bright green tint) to moisturize our hair. The same soap she used to bath us, she also used to wash our hair. We didn't have fancy shampoos and conditioners, and for medicinal purposes she used shea butter – a product I swear by, and use for my skin and hair, but which was largely unpopular, back then. I can still smell it today.

TIPS & TRICKS

Children's Afro haircare

I believe your child's haircare should be an enriching and healthy experience. These days, there are many products on offer, but hair maintenance for kids should be simple. Here are my haircare tips for children aged three and upwards.

Parents should use 1 or 2 applications of a mild shampoo (limited sulphates or parabens) followed by a moisturizing conditioner.

- A leave-in conditioner is advisable when combing the hair after conditioning.
- Use a wide toothcomb or paddle brush so your child feels the least amount of discomfort.
- During detangling, separate your child's hair into four or five sections with butterfly clips, then hold each section of hair by the base of the scalp and brush from the hair shaft up.
- Braids, cornrows, twists and even a light blow-dry are convenient for parents, and the protective styles are healthy for the hair. Avoid braiding or twisting too tightly.

- The scalps of children's hair are more sensitive and prone to irritation, burns and hair loss. I suggest staying away from chemicals until children are ready and able to take responsibility for the care and maintenance of their hair.
- Some parents decide to shave off babies' and infants' hair as it can help to promote abundance of growth and smoother texture, which can make hair manipulation easier. It is, of course, up to each parent, but many people have reported noticing the benefits of trimming hair in infancy. (Always check in with a medical practitioner first, and be sure to use a clean blade.)

NEW MUMS AND AFRO HAIRCARE

One of the amazing benefits of pregnancy is that many women experience an abundance of hair growth, with even more blood flow to the scalp, and a possible change in hair texture. The hormones secreted during this time often make hair stronger, healthier and shinier. Despite this, a woman's hair might shed as soon as she's given birth or starts to breastfeed. The stress of being a new mum, post-natal depression and fatigue can also contribute to hair loss. If possible, women with Afro hair should keep it natural and short during pregnancy. It's one of the easiest ways to guarantee that you'll stay looking incredible. Short haircuts can be low maintenance but still stylish and fun.

It's also advisable to avoid chemical treatments while pregnant, such as relaxers, Brazilian Blowouts and colouring. The scalp could potentially absorb the chemicals and affect the foetus, especially during the first trimester. I suggest indulging in more hair conditioning treatments during this time, but ones that are less heat-intensive. Pregnancy is the perfect time to leave the hair alone and indulge in a detox as the body goes through its hormonal changes.

HAIRSTYLES THROUGH THE AGES

Wigs

My Aunties Op, Diana and Vida were good at sewing and excellent dressmakers. The latter two were stay-at-home mums, while Auntie Op, the youngest and most carefree, travelled all over the continent for six months at a time, exporting cosmetics in bulk. She spent a lot of time in Lagos, Nigeria, in the 70s and 80s, when the country flourished and the naira was almost as strong as the pound. Auntie Op returned home from her trips with the latest relaxed looks, and I remember going with her to the local salons, which weren't exactly high-end compared to the salons of today but had modern appliances like ceiling fans, hair dryers and pressing combs. I'd look at the posters of all the different hairstyles you could have in those days, from traditional hair threading and relaxers to luxurious wigs. Adults, both men and women, experimented with wigs in the 70s, with my uncles sporting Afro wigs and my aunties wearing special pieces for occasions such as weddings or Christmas. I specifically remember chignons (more commonly referred to as buns) and beehives (big poofy hairdos) being very popular. Head coverings seemed to take over from more traditional hairdressing techniques, such as braiding and threading, and contributed hugely to the gradual disappearance of elaborate hair designs in African life.

There are many reasons why women and men decide to wear wigs – from wanting to make beauty statements to handling issues such as hair loss. For instance, women who wear their hair naturally still want versatility, which a wig can bring, and even more women want to move away from damaging chemical processes, or the glueing methods of weaves. Glamorous singers like Diana Ross were known to wear flamboyant pieces, and many entertainers and models wore wigs for work, play or as a protective style.

Wigs go way back. Head coverings made of synthetic or natural hair go as far back as Ancient Egypt (around 1150 BCE), where wigs were worn to disguise heads shaved bald for hygiene. Head lice were a concern in those days and thrived on the scalp's dense supply of blood vessels. Not only did wigs protect the head from the harsh effects of African sunlight (especially ageing), but they also allowed women to indulge quickly in new styles. Synthetic pieces were made from animals, including horses and sheep, and were often combined with plant fibres.[11] These were much cheaper than the human hairpieces coming from enslaved people, or those looking to make more capital, as human hair was just as valuable as gold. Only the upper classes could afford to wear wigs, as they were both expensive and time-consuming to make.

TIPS & TRICKS

Choosing the best wig

Contemporary wigs come in a variety of hair types, from human hair to synthetic, or a mix of both. Virgin hair and Remy hair are types of human hair that are one hundred per cent natural.

- **Virgin hair** comes from a living person and a single donor and has not been processed by any chemical treatments such as dyes or perms.
- **Remy hair**, on the other hand, has been chemically processed by the donor in the past. Human hair wigs allow for endless styling options and can be curled or straightened with heated appliances. They also offer a more natural texture and longer durability, depending on maintenance.
- **Synthetic wigs** (or a blend of human hair and synthetic) are the way to go if you're looking for a fuss-free wig with an already established style and cut. Some synthetic wigs cannot be curled or straightened using heated appliances, otherwise the hair would burn or melt. Budget is also something to consider when choosing a wig, as human hair options tend to be more expensive than synthetic.

On the high street, you can find synthetic wigs from as little as £25 (or $40), while professionally made wigs can cost anything from £400 to £1,500 ($500 to $2,600). You can also make your own wigs at home. Should you have the required skills for this, it

27

is preferable to do this yourself as it gives you flexibility with the shape and texture of the hair, and you can get a more natural look. However, if you do not have advance training in hair styling, it would be preferable to either collaborate with someone who does or opt for a pre-made wig.

These days, **lace front wigs** are all the rage. The sheer attachment at the front blends in with the hairline, giving the wig a more natural and believable look. Hair can be worn away from the face without revealing any demarcation line. Make sure wigs are made with a breathable net so that your scalp gets plenty of air, and avoid any methods requiring glue as this will destroy your hairline. When choosing a wig, consider the cut and also your face shape – if possible, try a short or mid-length wig. Wigs that are dated may make you look older than your years, so I would avoid these, as well as cuts that lack movement. Wigs can accentuate your best features, so here are a few tips and tricks for selecting the right head covering for your face shape:

- If you have good cheekbones, try a wig that accentuates and brings them out. Alternatively, wear a wig that softens your features. Try styles such as pixie cuts, bobs or tapered cuts.
- If you have a petite face, avoid wigs that are too big, or too curly or frizzy, as they will obscure your face. Opt for a sleeker wig that shows off your best assets. A graduated bob would suit an oval-shaped face.
- If you have an amazing jawline, do it justice! Go for a cropped style with added height on top to soften the face. Add definition to the curls so they don't frizz.
- Avoid wigs that look too much like wigs! Styles where the curls are too flat on top and too wide at the bottom might make your face look broader than it is.

Although synthetic fibres are cheaper, they often don't look the most natural or realistic to mimic our curl pattern, and they never last as long. Invest not only in a wig that mimics the true texture of Afro hair, but one that has been made for your head shape.

HOW TO MAINTAIN HAIR UNDERNEATH A WIG

Wigs are a way to change your look and to give your own hair a rest. They allow you to temporarily transform your look without compromising the health of your natural hair, making them the ultimate protective style. It's important to maintain the integrity and health of your natural hair beyond any protective style. Here are a few tips for taking care of your natural hair when wearing a wig.

- Wash your hair regularly. Think of your scalp the way you would think of your face. Would you go a month without washing it? Products and sweat cause build-up on the scalp, so hair should be washed with shampoo at least once a week.
- Spend some extra time deep conditioning your hair. Use rich conditioners and masks, as they repair and add shine to dull hair (skip to page 220 in Part 2 of this book for home-made mask recipes).

- Moisturize your hair and braid it underneath before applying the wig (any kind of thick braids or flat twists will do – with or without extension).
- Once the hair is braided, use an oil or serum to lightly coat the braids and to reduce friction and frizz caused by clips and wig caps.
- Avoid sleeping in a wig, to allow the follicles to breathe.

HOW TO MAINTAIN A WIG

Your hair

Regardless of the style you are rocking on top of your head, nothing is as crucial to hair health as keeping the scalp healthy and thriving. It's important to keep natural hair clean, fresh and moisturized underneath a wig. Try making a few rough braids or cornrows while you keep this style, and keep them for no more than two weeks.

Washing your wig

When washing your wig, use a moisturizing shampoo. Follow the steps below for the best results.

- Hold the wig in your hands and gently wet the hair with lukewarm water. Once the hair is thoroughly wet, apply a generous amount of shampoo, distributing evenly throughout.

- Rinse the wig under a stream of lukewarm water until all the shampoo is out. Remove the excess water by gently blotting with a towel.
- Apply conditioner, using your fingers to evenly distribute it throughout the hair.
- Rinse the wig under a stream of lukewarm water by gently patting and pressing with a soft towel. Use a paddle brush or a wide toothcomb and gently brush the hair, section by section.
- Blow-dry, scrunch-dry with a towel, or air-dry according to your desired style.
- **Note: Avoid heat for synthetic wigs, and use only a low heat on natural ones.**

Brushing/combing/scenting

If possible, be gentle while brushing, as you do not want to lose strands of hair. Comb or brush kindly, and use a non-greasy mist, otherwise you risk having to wash your wig regularly. If you are storing the wig in an enclosed space, try using some lavender in a pouch to give it a fresh scent.

HAIR LOSS

The importance of hair as a societal symbol of beauty is never so apparent as when a woman loses it. Hair loss is an emotional and traumatizing experience for many women, one that involves a journey towards acceptance and the regaining of self-confidence.

Alopecia is a condition related to hair loss or baldness on the scalp or any place on the body where hair grows. There are many different types of alopecia, including *alopecia areata*, which causes round, bald patches on the scalp or anywhere on the body, *alopecia totalis*, which affects the entirety of the scalp, and *alopecia universalis*, which includes all of the scalp and the body. Most forms of alopecia are caused by the immune system attacking the body – or, in this case, the hair follicles – preventing any sort of hair growth. There are also scarring and non-scarring types of alopecia. The latter means that the hair follicle is still protected, despite hair loss due to breakage or a change in the hair cycle, and the former means that the hair follicle is permanently damaged because of inflammation.

Traction alopecia is a type of non-scarring alopecia that is caused by excessive manipulation and styling, creating bald patches on the scalp. **Alopecia areata** is the most common form of hair loss and can be hereditary. The chance of hair growing back is slim, although not impossible, but this is also dependent on age and the location of the bald spots. Treatments such as steroid creams, injections and tablets are sometimes suggested by a doctor to help stimulate hair growth, but again, this depends on the severity.

There are clients who come to the Hair Lounge too ashamed to reveal their hair in public. They request to see me after hours or on my days off to ensure no other eyes are on them. I've even reserved private corners in the salon just to provide a sense of safety and to calm the anxiety and nerves of the client. Oftentimes, coming to the salon with hair loss can make a woman feel naked and exposed. Although hair loss can be hereditary, or due to menopause or stress, sometimes the cause boils down to inexperienced hairdressers who have braided hair too tightly or clients who have kept their braids in too long, all of which contributes to hair loss either around the hairline or on the crown of the head. Bonding glue applied to the scalp during a weave is also dangerous and can create bald patches, especially near the hairline, because the follicles are quite sensitive and need to be able to breathe.

In such instances, wigs are a great way for women to reclaim some power and self-esteem if dealing with hair loss and its emotionally crippling effects. The way I like to apply a wig is by putting a net over the head and then stitching the hair very softly so as not to disturb the rest of the hair. I tend to use a lot more hair than I would on other clients, in order to conceal the patches or bald spots. I like to finish the sew in with a nice cut that suits the client's face and brings out her features. Although the style is a temporary one, having the right hairdo can be a significant step in the journey towards a positive body image.

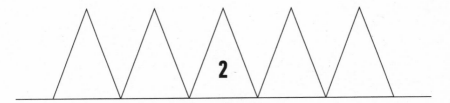

2

BACK TO BLACK

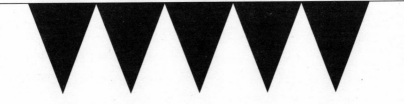

THE SCIENCE OF HAIR

Hair is truly one of the marvels of Blackness. Whether we celebrate the rhythm of our coils, or opt for straighter styles, our options are greater and more diverse than ever. I want to spend a little time discussing the basic science and composition of hair. If we know more about the structure of our hair, then we know how to take care of it. So, what are the basics you need to know?

The growth cycle

There are three phases to the human hair growth cycle:

- **Anagen** is the active phase of hair follicle growth where the hair grows for 1,000 days or more. *Hair follicles* are small holes all over the skin, including the scalp, that grow hair, and the *hair bulb* is at the base of the follicle where the hair is most alive and thriving until it passes through the scalp and dies.
- The **catagen** phase follows the active phase and involves the shrinkage of the hair follicles, where the hair becomes loosely attached. It's during this phase that hair loss occurs from the manipulation of brushing or combing, with about 100 hairs shedding per day. This phase lasts for up to two

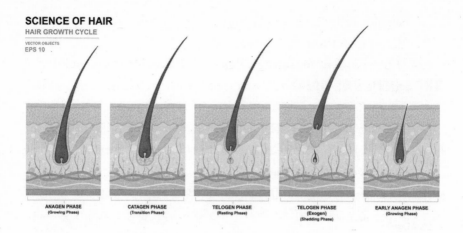

SCIENCE OF HAIR
HAIR GROWTH CYCLE

VECTOR OBJECTS
EPS 10

ANAGEN PHASE
(Growing Phase)

CATAGEN PHASE
(Transition Phase)

TELOGEN PHASE
(Resting Phase)

TELOGEN PHASE
(Exogen)
(Shedding Phase)

EARLY ANAGEN PHASE
(Growing Phase)

SHAPE OF THE HAIR

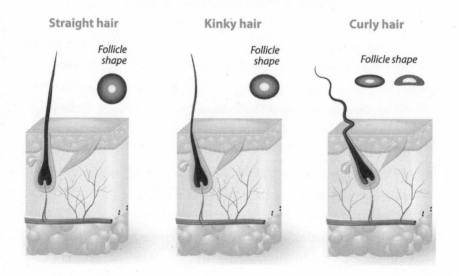

Straight hair

Follicle shape

Kinky hair

Follicle shape

Curly hair

Follicle shape

38

weeks and is a time when the hair follicles get ready to settle into their final phase.

- The **telogen** phase is the last of the hair growth cycle and is known as the resting phase, which lasts approximately 100 days. What makes Afro hair different from other types of hair is the shape of the hair follicle, which is often oval as opposed to circular, which produces straight hair.

The scalp

The scalp is the birthplace of the hair on our heads, and if kept in proper condition, it will provide the optimal environment for the follicles to produce quality locks. In order to grow hair that thrives, your scalp should remain clean, toned, pliable and stimulated.

The scalp, like the rest of the skin, is divided into three layers: the **epidermis** (uppermost), the **dermis** (middle) and the **subcutaneous** (bottom). The first layer acts as a protective surface and lacks blood vessels or nerves, while the third layer houses the scalp's very dense supply of blood vessels and fatty tissues. The middle layer contains collagen protein which lends strength and support to the skin. It's important to hydrate the body from within to fight scalp dryness. If you're dehydrated, your body will supply little moisture to the upper layers of your skin, and you'll then have to rely on external moisturizing products to hydrate your scalp. The healthy scalp produces an ounce of **sebum**, or oil, every

SKIN ANATOMY

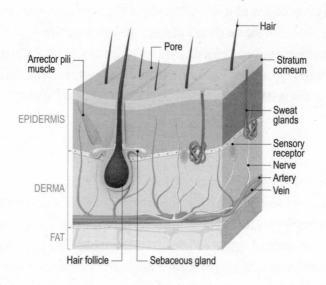

Hair

Pore

Arrector pili muscle

Stratum corneum

EPIDERMIS

Sweat glands

Sensory receptor

Nerve

Artery

Vein

DERMA

FAT

Hair follicle

Sebaceous gland

HAIR ANATOMY

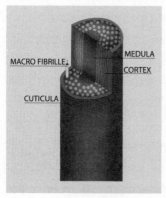

MACRO FIBRILLE

MEDULA

CORTEX

CUTICULA

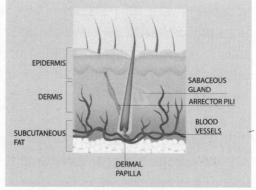

EPIDERMIS

DERMIS

SUBCUTANEOUS FAT

SABACEOUS GLAND

ARRECTOR PILI

BLOOD VESSELS

DERMAL PAPILLA

40

hundred days, and this comes from the natural breakdown of small cells within the **sebaceous glands**. Sebum's main job is to condition the skin and hair and act as a barrier to prevent internal moisture loss. The sebaceous glands are part of the hair follicle. These glands produce sebum, and our hair and skin's natural oil can be found on every part of the body except the palms of our hands and the soles of our feet.

The hair shaft

Lastly, there's the **hair shaft**, the part of your hair seen on the surface of the skin and scalp. It's composed of dead skin that's been transformed into a very strong protein called **keratin**, the same material that our nails are made of. Natural hair textures have 'an uneven build-up of keratin along the hair shaft; the hair bends where the keratin layers are heaviest and thins where they are less. This gives the movement along the hair shaft.'[1] The hair shaft is made of three layers: the **medulla** (the innermost layer, typically found in thicker hair), the **cortex** (found between the medulla and the cuticle – this is where hair strength, colour and elasticity originate) and the **cuticle** (the outermost layer, made of five to eleven overlapping sheaths, often described as looking like the shingles on a roof).

The healthy appearance of hair (and its glossiness) depends upon the condition of the cuticle, and harsh chemical treatments play a part in wearing away these protective layers. The cortex, on the other hand, is the most significant layer, making up the bulk of the hair. Afro and curly hair types have both a para and ortho cortex, which means that the structure of one side of a single hair differs from the other. 'The ortho cortex has a less dense structure and a lower sulphur content than the para cortex and always lies on the outside of the wave.'[2] This is why you feel different textures in your hair, and this is why we need to manipulate our hair more.

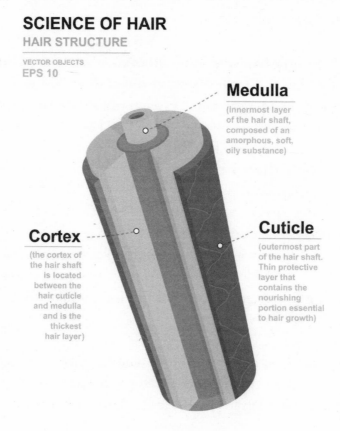

SCIENCE OF HAIR
HAIR STRUCTURE

VECTOR OBJECTS
EPS 10

Medulla

(innermost layer of the hair shaft, composed of an amorphous, soft, oily substance)

Cortex

(the cortex of the hair shaft is located between the hair cuticle and medulla and is the thickest hair layer)

Cuticle

(outermost part of the hair shaft. Thin protective layer that contains the nourishing portion essential to hair growth)

CURL TYPES

Curl types are a good blueprint for figuring out your routine curl pattern and to describe the shape of your curls. It's best to examine your curls whilst your hair is wet, as the texture is more evident and most people have several textures in their hair. Some people like to follow the curl type rules, as it's easier to know how to enhance their texture with the correct products.

The curl type system came from the curly community in America and was created as a useful guide, so you know where to start when it comes to haircare. In general, there are four types of

HAIR TYPES

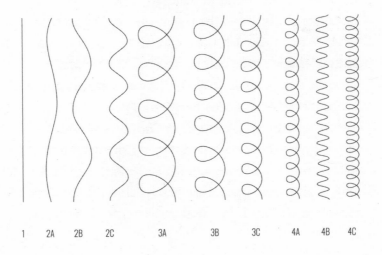

| 1 | 2A | 2B | 2C | 3A | 3B | 3C | 4A | 4B | 4C |

hair: straight, wavy, curly and kinky. Each type can be broken down into three subcategories, explained below.

For the purposes of this book, I start with kinky hair first and work my way back.

Kinky hair

Kinky hair is the hair type that most Black people have. This kind of hair is extremely wiry and has tight coils. It is also fragile and very prone to damage.

- Type 4A has a defined curl pattern almost like an S-shape. It retains moisture well but, as with most curly hair types, can still be prone to dryness.
- Type 4B hair is similar in shape to Type 4C – the only thing that changes between the two is the density and coarseness. Type 4B has a less definitive pattern of curl and looks more like a Z-shape as the hair bends at a sharp angle.
- Type 4C hair is tightly coiled in its raw state (meaning without products and just washed). There is no defined curl pattern and the coils must be defined by styles such as twisting, braiding, etc. Many Type 4C naturals have 70 per cent shrinkage or more and while the hair may be ten inches long, it gives the appearance of only about three inches unstretched. This is the most fragile of the hair types.

Curly hair

Curly hair has a clearly defined and springy shape and tends to be easy to style. The hair starts to get more prone to damage and is easily affected by the weather, such as rain or humidity.

- Type 3A hair has defined curls with a thick texture and a lot of shine but can be frizzy.
- Type 3B hair has tighter curls and may have a combination of textures.
- Type 3C hair has very tight curls or kinks and is generally easy to style.

Wavy hair

Wavy hair often becomes frizzy due to its mixed texture, between straight and curly.

- Type 2A hair has waves that are fine with a loose, tousled texture.
- Type 2B hair is mostly straight at the roots but falls into a more defined S-shape wave from mid-length to the end.
- Type 2C hair has waves that are more defined at the roots and ends with curls or ringlets. This texture is thicker and coarser and prone to frizzing.

Straight hair

Straight hair usually becomes greasy a lot faster than curly hair because oil from the scalp travels down the hair shaft more quickly. Straight hair tends to be the shiniest of all types and is also the strongest.

- Type 1A hair is very straight and fine. Most common in women of Asian descent.
- Type 1B hair is still very straight but is thicker with medium texture and more volume.
- Type 1C hair, while still straight, is very thick, coarse and shiny.

HAIR POROSITY

Hair porosity is the ability of the hair to absorb and keep moisture. It determines how well water, oils and moisturizing products penetrate the cuticle or the outermost layer of the hair. You can test the porosity of your hair by using a floating technique. Take a couple of strands of clean, dry hair (just shampooed) and drop them into a glass of water. If the strands float to the top of the glass before sinking, you have **low porosity hair**.

Women with Afro hair textures typically have low porosity hair, which makes it more difficult to keep the hair properly hydrated. Hair that takes longer to saturate when wet or takes a bit longer to dry are signs of low porosity. Products also tend to rest on low porosity hair, instead of being absorbed, making build-up more of an issue. If the strands sink to the bottom of the glass quickly, you have **high porosity hair**. Hair that hovers in between the top and bottom of the glass before eventually sinking indicates **medium porosity hair**.

TIPS & TRICKS

Tips for low porosity hair

You cannot change the porosity of your hair, because of genetics, but women with low porosity hair can do a few things for easier moisture absorption.

- Use protein-free conditioners, and apply conditioners when the hair is wet. Hair steamers or plastic caps during the conditioning phase of your wash are also recommended as this helps to penetrate the hair shaft.
- Use one hundred per cent shea butter (raw and unrefined) as a way to seal in moisture in combination with lightweight oils and products.
- Avoid excessive chemical treatments and heat from flat irons or blow-dryers as repeated use will make the hair even more porous.

AFRO HAIR MAINTENANCE

It's not that Type 4 hair is 'difficult' to maintain, it's just that it requires much more love and care in comparison to other types. Afro hair textures absorb liquid like a sponge, although the hair struggles to retain moisture, meaning our head tends to sweat a lot during the night, often leaving the hair dry and dull (hence why your pre-bed routine matters so much!). Women should see their haircare maintenance as a sacred time – after all, our hair has always been seen within Black communities as an expression of both creativity and spirituality. Below are several essential ways to look after Afro hair.

Washing

When caring for Afro hair, I always advise my clients to wash their hair weekly with a good-quality moisturizing shampoo that contains extra emollients (moisturizer) followed by a rinse-out conditioner. Products formulated for dry or damaged hair are the most nourishing.

Avoid fads like **co-washing** (using a conditioner to wash your hair), which creates build-up in the scalp, clogging the follicles and promoting hair loss. It's up to the individual how often you wash your hair. You'll usually know when the time is right, but once a week is a good indication.

Co-washing became popular in recent years as many users found that their shampoos were too harsh and left their scalps dry. In actual fact, co-washing is like getting in the shower and using a moisturizer instead of a skin cleanser. This is why it's essential to use the right shampoo. A good shampoo should have humectants that moisturize, a small amount of sulphates (which create the suds that cleanse) and, if possible, few parabens as this ingredient has been linked to hormonal problems.

I attended a hair loss clinic where a middle-aged Black woman visited. She had been co-washing for about twelve months as she wanted to use only natural products. The months of just co-washing had clogged her scalp, making it drier. The hair smelled of mildew and looked white as it had an accumulation of product. Because of the state of her scalp, the client had started to experience hair loss.

The most popular service at my Hair Lounge salon is a conditioning treatment and wash and blow-dry because without clean hair and a clean scalp, it is hard to style your hair or have any growth. It's important to shampoo and condition the hair on a regular basis to avoid dry, itchy scalp conditions such as dandruff caused by infrequent washing, fungal conditions, psoriasis, dry skin and sensitivity to hair products. If you suffer from any of these conditions, it's often a good idea to wash with a medicated shampoo or see your doctor for more advice.

Steaming

If you're looking to make potentially dry and brittle hair happy, why not steam your hair immediately after washing? Steaming is the process of using moist heat to help open the hair follicle. It also lifts the cuticle on the hair shaft, allowing conditioner and treatments to penetrate each strand of the hair and allowing for better absorption of moisture. It increases softness, stimulates growth and encourages blood flow.

After washing your hair with shampoo, apply a generous amount of conditioner to the hair, cover with a plastic cap and wrap with a hot towel or sit under a steamer for twenty to thirty minutes for the best results.

Steaming is one of the best things you can do to look after your hair as the heat aids in its hydration. Over time, hair will feel more manageable and will improve elasticity and moisture retention. I recommend steaming the hair every seven to ten days, especially for those who have colour-treated hair, low porosity hair, or who are transitioning hair from chemically relaxed to natural, as it softens the demarcation between the straight strands and the natural curls.

Detangling

Curly and Afro hair textures should always be detangled when wet and/or in combination with an oil or conditioner or a leave-in to help the process. Hair should also be divided into sections and then detangled section by section to aid in manageability. Starting at the bottom allows you to gently detangle each knot, rather than yanking your way through with a comb or brush, which can cause damage. I tend to use a paddle brush on curly and thick textured hair, which mimics the action of a wide toothcomb. Use a brush with bristles that don't have knots at the end so that it glides through the hair seamlessly without all the pulling and tugging.

Hot oil treatments

Practise regular hot oil treatments (with any type of oil that you like) to seal in moisture. Use a rehydrating and strengthening conditioning mask at least every two weeks, or once a month at a minimum. Treatments work best when heat is applied (under a steamer, for example), as this helps to open the hair cuticle and enables the nutrients to penetrate and nourish deeply within.

Trimming

Afro hair needs to be trimmed regularly, ideally every six to eight weeks, to ensure healthy ends and better curl definition. In the salon, we blow-dry the hair first (using low heat) before trimming to achieve a straighter and more accurate cut.

Scalp massage

Try and give your scalp a one-minute massage each day using small, clockwise motions of the fingers. The better your scalp circulation, the stronger the 'power supply' is to your hair follicle, so you'll have less hair falling out. This simple practice stimulates the secretion of sebaceous oils and stimulates blood circulation.

Heat protection

If you must use heat when styling, always use a heat protection as Afro hair is more prone to breakage than any other hair type. Drying methods include air-drying, hood-drying or blow-drying with a diffuser. Try using serums, oils and pomades with an advanced level of silicone, which acts as a coating that helps to protect hair.

Hair breaks

You're unlikely to experience significant hair growth if you don't give your hair a break. Try wrapping your hair once a week for the day, if you can, to give it a break from styling. In between protective styles, try to give yourself one or two weeks without a style, so that your scalp can rest and your hair can have the benefit of sufficient natural oils before experiencing any further hair tension. Keep the ritual fun and look for beautiful prints. Centre the material at the nape of your neck, bringing both ends to the front. Criss-cross, then wrap around to the back and knot.

Night-time rituals

Take five minutes to pamper your hair before bedtime. That means moisturizing, if necessary, and securing the ends with a silk or silk-satin scarf. I like to use a silk wrap, because I find the cotton pillowcase can draw moisture out of the hair. If you don't have access to silk, it's okay to use a synthetic fabric with a silky finish – it can cost anything from £3 to £25.

Product cocktails

Product cocktailing is simply mixing two or three products together to meet your specific styling needs. My favourite cocktail is curl cream (a moisturizer and hydrater which adds definition to your hair) with a tiny amount of styling gel and some Manketti Oil. This allows for a supreme hold without leaving your hair dry and crunchy.

Oils

Most Afro hair soaks up moisture like a sponge, so seal in moisture using natural oils. Another reason to use oils, especially on the scalp area, is if you suffer from a dry and itchy scalp, which often worsens in the winter. An excellent tip for those who suffer from dandruff is to massage a good natural oil into the scalp and let it sit for twenty minutes before shampooing and conditioning thoroughly.

TIPS & TRICKS

What oils can I use for my hair?

When the scalp doesn't produce enough sebum on the hair shaft, hair oils can be used to supplement this deficiency. Natural hair oils are usually derived from plants and flowers and are used to lubricate, stimulate and keep moisture in the scalp. Many are rich in vitamins, minerals, fatty acids and proteins. To help stimulate blood flow, massage oils in a circular motion into a clean scalp once or twice a week, as needed. It's important to note that oils on their own do not moisturize natural hair – rather, they act as sealants – so it's best to supplement a good oil with a butter, along with moisturizing shampoos and conditioners. Besides my Manketti Oil, which includes a cocktail of oils from argan to shea butter, making it rich, there are many other oils out there that can be used for a variety of purposes.

My advice when it comes to hair oils is to experiment. Concoct your own mixtures and see how your hair responds – all heads of hair are different, and what works for one person will not work for all. Some women might decide to opt for products created in a laboratory, rather than play around with natural ingredients. Whatever you decide, here are some general facts about oils and home ingredients, what they contain and what they may be used for.

- **Argan oil** is very popular now and is great for combating frizziness and adding a lustrous shine. Derived from the kernels of the argan plant, which is often used for drizzling on pasta, couscous or to dip in bread, it is a native product from Morocco. As such, one hundred per cent Moroccan varieties are best.
- **Coconut oil** is one of the few oils that help to penetrate the hair shaft instead of simply sealing in moisture. It's rich in monounsaturated fatty acids and full of vitamin E. Monounsaturated fatty acids are important because they penetrate deeper into the hair shaft and don't sit on top of the hair like other fatty acids. It's possible to buy coconut oil in most supermarkets, but make sure you use oil that is made for hair use.
- **Avocado oil** is excellent for protecting the hair against damage, making the hair feel soft and smooth due to its thick consistency. It also contains more monounsaturated acids than coconut oil. This oil is rich in many vitamins and minerals.
- **Black Jamaican castor oil** is a popular type of castor oil, derived from castor beans, which grow on the ricinus plant in tropical countries. It is thick and syrupy and can potentially regrow the hair, especially thin or damaged edges. It contains unsaturated fatty acids and other wonderful nutrients and minerals. It's also known for its antifungal and antibacterial properties.

Less is more with this oil as it can quickly clog up the scalp.

- **Extra virgin olive oil** is less processed than the rest of the olive oil family, therefore retaining much of its essential nutrients. It's an excellent oil to use for a dry and itchy scalp and for conditioning the hair as it works wonders for penetrating the hair shaft. It is high in monounsaturated fatty acids and antioxidants. Look out for any products that use extra virgin olive oil. If you find a high-quality olive oil, it is worth purchasing and using it for home-made preparations.
- **Jojoba oil** stimulates the scalp to create more sebum and is similar to olive oil in its molecular structure, making it an excellent oil for dry scalps.
- **Almond oil** is lightweight and smells particularly sweet and delicious. It works as an excellent sealant, making it perfect to use as a finisher after styling hair (for example, a mist or sheen spray).

PROTECTIVE STYLES

Protective styles are a good way to protect your hair from frequent manipulation. They help to prevent excessive breakage and promote length retention. Most of us use protective styles to grow or transition our hair or to take a break from combing and styling. Afro hair requires as little manipulation as possible, due to its fragility, and there are a multitude of protective styles out there that allow the hair to grow undisturbed with as little breakage as possible, including African hair threading, cornrowing, Bantu knots and twist outs.

TIPS & TRICKS

Basic Afro care

The LOC method

This is your go-to routine for your natural hair, on a daily or regular basis. (This is a trial and error process – be careful with putting too much on and clogging your pores!)

- Liquid/Leave-in – after washing or wetting your hair with a spray bottle, use a leave-in conditioner.
- Oil – from the list above, choose an oil that will nourish your hair. This is to seal in the water.
- Cream – use a moisturizing cream or pomade that will help to shape and define your curls. (Head to page 215 for cream recommendations.)

HAIRSTYLES THROUGH THE AGES

African hair threading

I remember hair threading being very popular when I was growing up in Ghana in the 70s. The same aunties who used to wear wigs would also have their hair threaded by a deaf family friend named Mumiiu who was an expert with her fingers. As a child, I used to watch her shape the individually threaded strands into baskets on top of the head, tie them back into a bun or allow the strands to hang around the face, depending on how long the hair was. She also etched various patterns and shapes, such as triangles and stars, into the scalp through the sectioning of the hair.

Hair threading involves wrapping wool, nylon or yarn around sections of partitioned hair, tightly and evenly. The hair becomes stiff but easy to manipulate into intricate geometric shapes that sit on top of the head. Indigenous to many parts of Africa, the hairdo is an excellent example of the way hair has been used as adornment. Hair threading also illustrates how Afro hair lends itself to sculpting techniques due to its thickness and texture.

A TALE OF CULTURAL DIFFERENCES

In 1981, I moved from the tropical climate of Ghana to the concrete jungle known as Stonebridge in North West London, at the age of eleven, to return to my parents. The only image I had then of the city came from the Peter and Jane books I'd read as a child. Whenever my grandparents spoke to me of London, it seemed like a fairytale place and I couldn't wait to arrive. But now it seemed my old world of light, love and laughter had been replaced with cold and unhappy faces. I waited at Heathrow with my guardians until one of my parents, who were no longer together, could pick me up. Mum and Dad had visited my siblings and me in Ghana throughout the years, but this would be my first time living with either one of them. Dad came in the evening and drove me home to see Mum and my three siblings, but as soon as we arrived all I could think was, 'Oh no, I want to go back to Ghana!'

Life on the council estate was not like the large compound I'd grown up on. I now lived in a council house on a blacklisted estate. As soon as you said the words 'Stonebridge' people automatically said, 'Oh, you live in that bad area?' The neighbourhood was notorious for its gang culture, it was deemed so bad that you couldn't even get a store catalogue delivered to your door. The media often painted the area in a bad light, but growing up there felt completely different to what we heard about in the news. People generally looked after each other and I felt safe, but the two worlds were like chalk and cheese. London was too quiet, and even though I lived in a place with amenities like electricity, a modern kitchen and a TV, I missed the way Mama lit the lanterns at night as soon as it got dark. My refrain of 'Oh, I want to go back to Ghana' must have driven my mum mad. She'd always respond with 'Okay, if you want to go back, I'll send you back' but of course she never did. It took a while to adjust to her, and to my new surroundings, as I'd missed out on the formative years of our relationship.

I spent three months, from November to January, helping Mum around the house. School was already in full swing, so I had to wait until the new year to attend. I pushed my sister's pram whenever Mum took her to nursery, and contributed to chores around the house. Mum liked everything clean, making me tidy about ten times before she became satisfied. I loved organizing her room, paying special attention to her vanity unit where she kept a lot of the fragrances, powders and creams she had as an Avon lady, one of her many odd jobs besides cleaning. She used to say to me, 'Come on. Let's go round and knock on the doors,' and together we'd go and see who would buy the products. Eventually, I took over myself, packing the orders when they came in and collecting the money afterwards.

Mum wore voluminous Afro wigs, back in the day, and loved dressing up and looking nice. We always watched soaps together like *Dallas* or *Dynasty*, and every week I looked forward to seeing Alexis Carrington on screen. I saw a lot of Mum's loneliness in those days. She was a woman on her own trying to raise three kids while juggling a handful of jobs. Apart from supporting her children (there were eight of us living between Ghana and London by the time she was thirty-nine), she worked hard to send money back home. It took a lot of integrity and a lot of strength to raise us on her own, but she was no-nonsense and often did what she had to do. I think a lot of my independence comes from that.

Dad would visit once a week, on a Sunday, from Queen's Park, nearby. Dad was very charismatic and probably had one too many friends. He worked for the London Underground as a tube driver at the time and no longer worked at the Grosvenor House Hotel. Mum liked to dress us in our Sunday best whenever he came to visit, and in those days girls wore rara skirts in the summer or stonewashed denim jackets, ruffled blouses and stirrup leggings in the autumn. Dad usually took us to the Odeon on Edgware Road where we saw films like *Return of the Jedi* or *The Fox and the Hound*, but one of the reasons I loved him coming around the most was the Bargain Bucket from KFC he brought with him for lunch. It was a nice change from the home-cooked meals Mum made during the week. Mum and Dad were still very close then and I loved listening to their conversations. I used to think to myself, 'Why don't they just get back together?' because they seemed to get on so well. They could spend hours on the phone just laughing and talking about all sorts of things, but unfortunately, they weren't meant to be.

The new year came around, and Mum finally found me a school to attend. I was looking forward to going back because I'd been popular at Harrow International and excelled at all my exams. When it came to algebra and arithmetic, I knew all my times tables, decimal points and fractions. I also had an excellent understanding of the English language. So, walking into Copeland

High School in Wembley on the 5th of January 1982 was a shock to the system. I felt as if I was walking into a United Colors of Benetton ad. It was unusual for me to be around kids who were Asian, West Indian or white. I had assumed they would all look like me, just as they had done in Ghana. Not only did the kids look different, they also called teachers by their first name, and made fun of them behind their backs or to their face. But the biggest surprise was the amount of bullying I faced as soon as I arrived. I seemed to be an alien from another planet whose dark skin, short hair and Ghanaian accent became the butt of every joke. I went from a place where people were very friendly and hospitable to the opposite, where the kids at Copeland chanted, 'Where are you from? You're an African boo-boo . . . say that again? You're an alien!'

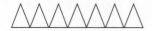

I seemed to be an alien from another planet whose dark skin, short hair and Ghanaian accent became the butt of every joke. I went from a place where people were very friendly and hospitable to the opposite, where the kids at Copeland chanted, 'Where are you from? You're an African boo-boo . . . say that again? You're an alien!'

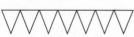

The day Mum sent me to school in a threaded hairstyle was probably the worst day of my life and the shapes on top of my head were just another confirmation of my extra-terrestrial status. Girls at Copeland were sporting cornrows and relaxers, with hair pushed back into sleek ponytails. Even on TV, women like Diahann Carroll from *Dynasty* and stars from *Hotel* and *The*

Cosby Show had hair that was relaxed and styled into a bouncy look, blow-dried and full. It wasn't just the kids who laughed at my threaded hair but also the Jamaicans down in Harlesden, who used to turn their heads when Mum sent me to the shop for fruit and veg. I found it hard adjusting to the culture shock of being in England, and often came home in tears. Little did I know that one day I'd be responsible for bringing the style back on to the map. If you're feeling bold, the next section shows you how to create your own threaded look and explains the benefits of the ancient style.

Hair threading

Average styling time: 1 hour 30 minutes

Style duration: 1 to 2 weeks

Hair threading attracts much admiration but also controversy and, unfortunately, the style is dying out in Africa due to the popularity of more modern styles like braiding, relaxers and weaves.

I remember doing a feature on threading for *Black Beauty & Hair Magazine* in August/September 2009, where the reactions to the models were staggering. I never thought in a million years that my own people had forgotten the art of threading and that they would feel so averse to it. Onlookers thought that a contemporary woman wearing thread in her hair was daring or brave, while others felt it was a 'primitive' and 'uncivilized' thing to do. An older man said, 'Wow, it's been a long time since I've seen this kind of hairstyle. It reminds me of the good old days.'[3]

Threading is a great heat-free blow-dry as it stretches the hair, allowing it to grow long and soft. It offers the perfect balance between aesthetic and style. I remember once a young model/actress in her late twenties who came to the salon looking for a style for the upcoming season. Surprisingly, she'd heard about hair threading and wanted to give it a try, and from the get-go, I could tell she had an adventurous style and didn't mind standing out in a crowd. Threading is easier if you have someone else doing it for you, so grab a friend or head to the salon to get it done!

TIPS & TRICKS

How to thread hair

Here is a step-by-step guide to creating a simple threaded look.

Tools you will need

- Essential oil or other treatment (optional)
- Tail comb
- Paddle brush
- Black or coloured thread

Step by step

Only wash and style hair on the same day if you are doing a treatment. If not, give your hair at least five days of rest after shampooing and conditioning, then skip straight to Step 4.

1. Do a treatment first if you can. Separate the hair into four equal parts and apply an essential oil on the scalp. Allow to penetrate for fifteen minutes.
2. Rinse the hair thoroughly before you shampoo and condition. Towel dry and then apply one or two drops of oil.
3. Blow-dry the hair and brush out with a paddle brush or leave the hair to air-dry. You can also thread the hair while damp.
4. Divide the hair into eight sections.
5. Take one metre of shiny black or coloured thread in your dominant hand.
6. Hold one section of hair firmly at the scalp between your left thumb and forefinger and anchor the end of the thread by twisting it around the hair at the scalp.
7. Wind the thread clockwise around the section of hair and work your way up towards the end.
8. Once finished, knot the thread securely two or three times to avoid unravelling.
9. Repeat the same process with the other parted sections.

Hair can be threaded for up to two weeks before unwrapping, washing and conditioning. In terms of keeping the hair neat, wrap your hair with a silk scarf before bedtime, and to flatten flyaway strands use a flat-style natural bristle brush to keep the hairline smooth.

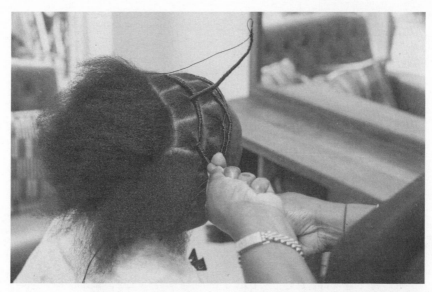

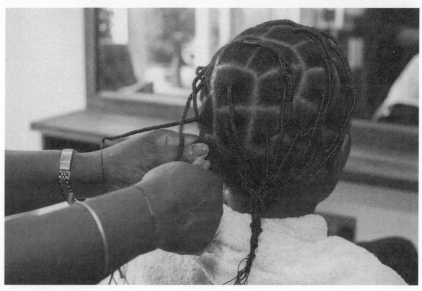

Cornrows

Average styling time: 2 to 3 hours

Style duration: 2 weeks maximum

Cornrows are another, more modern-day protective style using a three-strand braiding technique attached to the scalp in rows. They are an ancient African form of hair expression, memorialized in sculptures and hieroglyphics as far back as 500 BCE.[4] Author Victoria Sherrow writes that the Temne and Yoruba tribes in Africa spent hours upon hours engaging in the style, which they used as both an art form and for practical reasons during celebrations. Enslaved people in the American South wore cornrows to keep hair away from the face during labour in the fields. It is believed that Americans use the word 'cornrows' because it reminds them of cornfields, whereas in the Caribbean, the hairstyle is called 'canerows' because they resemble sugar cane.[5] Throughout the 60s and 70s, from the Black Power Movement onwards, many celebrities and musicians rocked cornrows as a way of reclaiming or paying respect to African roots, or as a form of rebellion against ideas of the style being urban or unprofessional. Like the Afro, cornrows took on a symbolic meaning and forward-thinking women like Nina Simone and Cicely Tyson were known to wear the look. Alicia Keys brought the style back into the limelight in the 90s and early 2000s, with her creative Fulani styles. Cornrows have had their fair share of controversy as non-Black men and women adopted the ancient style, from Bo

Derek in the 70s to David Beckham in 2003. It's one of a handful of Afro hairstyles that have been culturally appropriated, with a wide variety of opinions on the matter.

TIPS & TRICKS

Cornrowing

If you're looking to try the iconic style yourself, here is a step-by-step guide.

Tools you will need

- Tail comb
- Wide toothcomb
- Hair clips
- Hair bands
- Finishing mist or sheen spray

Step by step

Only wash and style hair on the same day if you are doing a treatment. If not, give your hair at least five days of rest after shampooing and conditioning, then start at Step 2.

1. Start with freshly prepped hair that has been shampooed, conditioned and moisturized.

2. Section the hair into your desired pattern, width or style with a wide toothcomb. How many rows do you want? Do you want them large or small? Will you braid from front to back or try something more complicated? Make sure your sections are evenly spaced out so that your rows are about the same size.

3. Use clips to secure each section before braiding. Alternatively, part your sections as you go and clip the rest of the hair back and out of the way.

4. Take a row of hair from the forehead and separate it into three further sections for braiding, gathering one section of hair in one hand, and two sections of hair in the other.

5. Move the right or left section over and on top of the centre section.

6. Move the section on the opposite side over.

7. Take the centre section and switch. Remember that the middle section of hair will always be the moving piece that travels from left to right. Always ensure that you have one section in one hand and two in the other, incorporating a small section of hair as you move along until you reach the nape of the neck (making sure the braid is attached to the head instead of loose).

8. Finish off the braid, depending on how long the hair is, and secure with a band.

9. Repeat with the other rows.

10. Use a light sheen spray or finishing mist for moisture.

Cornrows should not be applied too tightly and should not be kept in for longer than a couple of weeks. Make sure to continually oil the scalp while wearing the style.

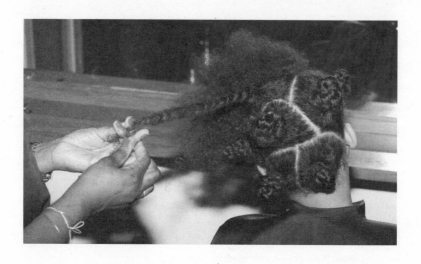

Bantu knots

Average styling time: 2 hours

Style duration : 1 week

Bantu knots are individual braids or twisted hair that's spun around itself to form a tight knot or coil. The protective style is thought to go as far back as 1898.[6] Although the word 'Bantu' describes hundreds of ethnic groups across Southern Africa, it's the Zulu who originally wore the look, thus the style can also be referred to as Zulu knots. It is also sometimes called Nubian knots (referring to a former region of Northern and Eastern Africa).

This style is amazingly simple to achieve but leaves the wearer looking regal. The beauty of a natural, free style such as Bantu knots is that you can go a week or two without having to shampoo, condition or apply products daily. Women who have thicker and longer natural hair can also leave the knots in overnight and remove them the next day to create voluptuous curls. Bantu knots are versatile and can be worn in a variety of ways, so get creative!

TIPS & TRICKS

How to do Bantu knots

Tools you will need

- Moisturizing butter or essential oil
- Tail comb
- Wide toothcomb
- Hairpins

Step by step

1. Shampoo and condition the hair as normal.
2. Apply a moisturizing butter or oil to damp hair and detangle.

3. Section the hair into small (for shorter hair) or big (for longer hair) shapes such as squares or triangles. The look illustrated here was sectioned into three horizontal squares around the head. Then, from the nape of the neck, triangle sections were parted from each square.

4. Take each section from the base and twist in one direction (or you can decide to opt for braids). I achieved the look by braiding each triangular section.

5. Wrap each twist or braid around itself at the scalp so that it forms a knot.

6. Use a hairpin to secure the end at the base, or tuck the end into the middle.

7. Continue the braiding, twisting and pinning throughout the entire head.

8. Apply a small amount of finishing pomade, butter or oil to the palms of the hand to straighten and smooth down the edges.

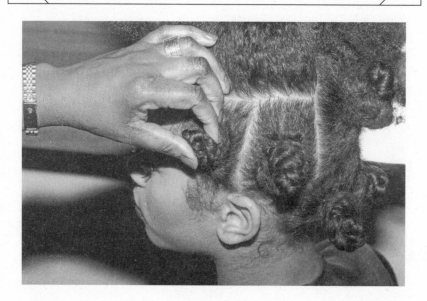

Twist outs

Average styling time: 1 hour 30 minutes

(Jumbo: 1 hour / Medium: 2 hours / Small: 3 hours)

Style duration: 1 to 2 weeks

Twist outs are incredibly easy to achieve – much more so than corn-rows, threading and Bantu knots. The style is a good way to detangle your hair at night while sleeping and can also be used afterwards as its own style, which creates beautiful S-shaped curls once dry. A good twist out seals moisture into the hair after shampooing and conditioning, especially when using a leave-in conditioner, butters or oils.

TIPS & TRICKS

How to do twist outs

Tools you will need

- Tail comb
- Wide toothcomb
- Leave-in conditioner
- Water

Step by step

1. Shampoo and condition the hair as normal.
2. Section the hair as desired.
3. Mix up two pumps (depending on hair length) of a rich leave-in conditioner and water, or cream, butter or pomade. Put into a spray bottle and moisturize the hair, section by section.
4. Take each section of damp hair and separate into two.
5. Start at the roots and twist each section around the other, winding as tightly as possible but not too tight.
6. Once at the end, twirl the tips of the hair around your fingers to prevent unravelling.
7. If preparing for bed, sleep with a silk or satin scarf or pillowcase to further seal in moisture.
8. Unravel the twists in the morning (or once fully dry) for beautiful S-shaped curls. Pick apart with the fingers for your desired look.

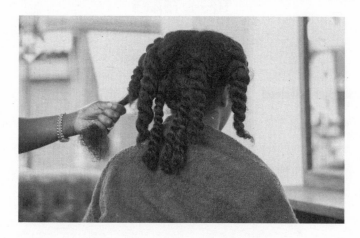

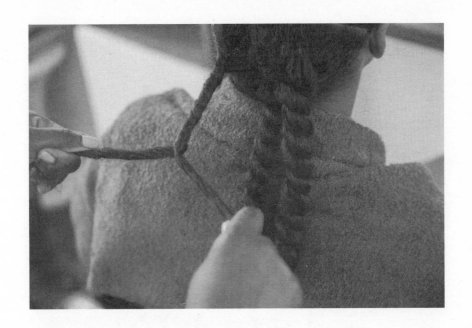

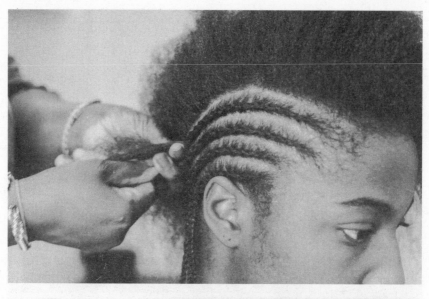

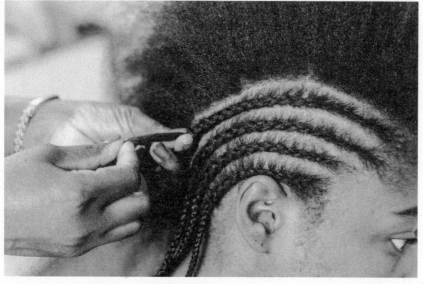

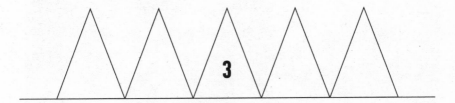

3

MOVING ON

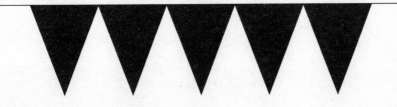

MUSIC TO HEAL THE BLUES

I have nice memories of having my hair pressed by my mother or eldest sister, Sheila. I remember large tubs of Dax grease, and the hot comb coming off the stove to give me that slicked-back pony-tail look. Of course, like most women and girls, I was never completely happy with the hair I had and spent a lot of time wishing my hair could be as long as that of the girls at school who could style their hair in cornrows. Every time they walked, the beads at the ends of the braids would click and clack.

Unfortunately, my own hair wasn't long enough to achieve such fun and colourful styles, and one of the things I disliked most about the hot comb was that once my hair got wet that was the end of the style and my hair would coil back to normal. Luckily for me, on my fourteenth birthday, my Auntie Janet took me to her local salon to experience my first curly perm. My hair was put into little rods, and how curly and smooth it looked afterwards! I loved my new look, despite having to sleep with a plastic cap every night (otherwise the activator drenched my pillows).

My new curly perm gave me little comfort, though, as the weeks and months before had been the hardest of my life. The past two years at Copeland High School had been calmer, and being in

London seemed a bit more manageable now, but things at home took an unexpected turn when I came home in April of 1983 to Mum having one of her headaches. Mum worried a lot and shouldered loads of responsibility, assuming the role of both matriarch and patriarch of our household. Naturally, this accentuated ailments, namely her high blood pressure. When she collapsed that afternoon, my brother and I called an ambulance. When we arrived at the hospital, we discovered her blood pressure was higher than normal, and so they kept her in for several days to run tests. My brother and I visited her after school for about ten days, but each day her health seemed to deteriorate. She lost her memory and after the results came through the doctors told us she had suffered a brain haemorrhage and that they would need to operate. The day before the operation they shaved off part of her hair, but suddenly, and inexplicably, she passed away. Just like that. Sometimes, I still relive that moment. Even when I think about it now, it's hard to process, as if it were still a bad dream. She died on the 16th of May 1983, six days before my thirteenth birthday, and my world changed forever after that.

My brother, sisters and I remained in the council house in Stonebridge for some time before we all went to live with my father in Queen's Park and then eventually Edmonton. Even though I had initially struggled, I'd made some really good friends in the neighbourhood since coming from Ghana, but now I would have to leave. I still went to Copeland High School in Wembley, but the bus journey from Queen's Park to Wembley was long, and

I filled my hours with music from a Walkman my father bought me. Music became my medicine, both speaking to and soothing my grief. I also discovered a lot of American artists like the Fatback Band, Loose Ends and the Jackson 5, Cherrelle and the S.O.S. Band and Evelyn 'Champagne' King, who had more of a soul flavour. My tastes were eclectic, and I loved a lot of the stuff my mum or my friends listened to on records, like Marvin Gaye (I still remember the day his father shot him dead, because I knew how much Mum loved him), Bob Marley (Mum cried and cried when he passed) and Chaka Khan, Tina Turner and Stevie Wonder.

I spent a lot of time in my room listening to music on pirate stations on Kiss FM, Horizon Radio and JVC or doing my younger sister's hair, just to make myself feel better. Mum used to love caring for her hair and now I felt I needed to carry on the tradition. I experienced a lot of grief in those days but the ritual of looking at lifestyle magazines like *Essence, Black Beauty & Hair, Ebony* and *Jet* and learning new hairstyles provided much solace. I copied the looks and used my sister as a model, and most of the dos consisted of cornrows which were popular at the time. I tasked myself with challenges such as braiding patterns on the scalp or applying beads at the end, which I always found difficult. After shampooing and conditioning her hair, I applied a bit of Dax, and then threaded her hair to straighten it out until braiding it the next day. We used to talk to each other during that time and I'd ask her about nursery and her new friends. Sometimes we spoke about Mum, but she was too young to understand what had happened and believed that Mum would be back. I told her Mum had gone to a better place, that she had gone up to heaven, but my brother knew better because sometimes he'd sit in the corner of the living room and cry. When I look back on it now, my passion for styling really began in the days, months and years following Mum's death. The braiding and learning gave me a sense of relief and a temporary joy. I enjoyed witnessing how cute my sister looked and recognizing my achievement for the day. Honestly, I don't know where I'd be today if I hadn't turned to hair for help.

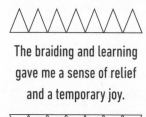

The braiding and learning gave me a sense of relief and a temporary joy.

HAIRSTYLES THROUGH THE AGES

Hot combs

The authors Phillip and Lesley Hatton write that African enslaved people used a variety of early hair straightening techniques, ranging from heated metal rods passed over the hair to pieces of cloth first wrapped around the locks and pressed with a heated can. It wasn't until 1872 that the first hot iron came into existence, when a French hairdresser named Marcel Grateau created the tool to put waves in European hair. The Marcel Wave became popular in the 1920s and 30s with entertainers like Josephine Baker (an African American singer, dancer and civil-rights activist living in France) adopting the style on her short, cropped hair. The hot iron later made its way to the States, where it was sold in department stores. It was later modified and made popular for an African American audience. It was heated over a stove or flame and then passed through Afro hair from the roots, over and over again, until straight. Although these combs were popular, they were dangerous due to the heated metal, making it easy to burn and damage the scalp. The combs also caused dryness and brittleness to the hair after long-term use, due to excessive heat. The hot comb made a comeback in the 80s but was never destined to last as an efficient way to straighten Afro hair as the style would immediately revert back to its kinky state once wet.

TIPS & TRICKS

Silk press

Average styling time: 2 to 3 hours, depending on hair length

Style duration: 2 to 4 weeks

The silk press process uses flat irons to straighten the hair and has replaced the outdated hot comb. Instead of heating a comb on the stove, a flat iron (an electric tool made of ceramic or metal plates) completes the look. It offers a cheaper and faster way to straighten the hair and can easily be done at home.

Step by step

1. After the hair is washed and conditioned with a moisturizing shampoo and conditioner, detangle the hair and blow-dry.

   It's always advisable to apply a heat protectant to the hair, which creates a barrier and helps protect it from the adverse effects of heat. Protectants come in creams, serums, sprays and oils and usually contain ingredients like silicones, amino acids and humectants – check out the label.

2. Once the hair is dry, divide the hair into sections panel by panel and pass the flat iron over each section (making sure the iron is half an inch away from the scalp) until the entire head is done.

   One pass using moderate heat is often enough (anything more than one or two passes is not advised). As with all heated appliances, less is more, as heat is damaging to the hair over a period of time.

Flat irons should not be used for hair that's relaxed or transitioning, as the hair is already straight and weakened by chemicals, making it more prone to breakage. Similar to the hot comb, you should avoid rain and humidity after pressing the hair, otherwise it will revert back to its kinky state. Flat irons should be used sparingly, as continued and excessive heat will ultimately weaken and destroy the integrity of the hair.

A silk press can last up to two weeks if normal haircare rules are applied, such as sleeping with a silk scarf, wrapping the hair up at night around the head, and using a plastic cap to protect the hair from moisture when showering.

KERATIN HAIR TREATMENTS

Brazilian Blowouts

Keratin treatments are a temporary way to make curly or frizzy hair more manageable, straight and sleek. They are also known as Brazilian Blowouts. These treatments are known to make dry and damaged hair look and feel stronger and healthier because of the infusion and restoration of the proteins (keratin) found in the hair, which are usually stripped away over time due to factors like age and chemical treatments.

Keratin treatments are usually a mix of keratin and other natural proteins like wheat and soy, but the proteins are also blended with inorganic ingredients. (Formaldehyde used to be an active ingredient before the realization of its toxicity.) A serum is applied to sections of freshly washed hair, and then steamed or blow-dried for the treatment to penetrate. Afterwards, the hair is rinsed, dried and straightened with an iron to seal the treatment into the hair. The process can take two to four hours, depending on the length and texture of the hair. Clients are advised not to wash the hair for forty-eight hours after the treatment in order to keep the hair straight and smooth. Any sort of manipulation of the hair, including styling and tying up, should also be avoided in that time. (Different treatments have different rules, so consult your stylist for more information.)

When washing your hair, use shampoos and conditioners that do not contain sulphates as these will break down the keratin in the hair. Your tresses will bounce back to their natural texture once washed, but after straightening you should notice a smoother, sleeker and shinier look. Rain and humidity won't affect the hair while the treatment is still in effect, which can last anywhere between two and five months, depending on hair type. After this time, the keratin will break down and the hair will revert back to its natural state.

What is keratin?

One of the most important components of human hair is a thread-like protein called keratin, which is a combination of organic compounds including carbon, oxygen, hydrogen and nitrogen. Keratin also contains sulphur, the principal compound that makes it possible for us to chemically straighten our hair. Keratin is made up of amino acids which are joined together by peptide bonds. The combination of amino acids and peptide bonds produces polypeptides, meaning more than one peptide bond. In human hair, polypeptides are cross-linked by other bonds. It's this innumerable set of linkages that makes the structure of our hair so complex. Keratin contains three types of cross-linkages, one of which is called a disulphide bond. When our hair is altered through chemical straightening, these are the bonds that are broken. They are the strongest of the three bonds and can only be broken down by chemicals.

HAIRSTYLES THROUGH THE AGES

Curly perms

The curly permanent (or Jheri curl) was a short-lived but popular hairstyle in the 80s for both Black men and women who wanted looser, softer and shinier curls. It was a variation of the permanent wave, a process primarily used for men and women with thick European hair. Permanents or 'perms' (which change the structure of the hair shaft from curly to straight or from kinky/coily to looser waves/curls, depending on the chemical and treatment) were first applied in the 1900s using electric machines and were later replaced with chemical cold creams. The curly permanent involved a multi-step process.

First, a cream (containing a salt called ammonium thioglycolate) was applied to straighten the hair. After a short period of time, the cream was rinsed off to stop the chemical process. A curl booster was added to the hair, which was then set in perm rollers with a neutralizer applied to lock the curls in place. According to stylists and authors Phillip and Lesley Hatton, neutralizers often contained oxidizing agents like hydrogen peroxide, which allowed the broken-down disulphide bonds in the keratin layer of the hair to re-form around the rollers, giving the hair a new shape. They also contained acids to get rid of any alkali components left from the cream. Maintenance of the style included spraying the hair every night with an activator to ensure the hair stayed moisturized and soft.

There are several chemists and hairdressers responsible for the rise of the curly perm. The first man, and its namesake, Jheri Redding, was an American businessman born in Illinois in 1902. He was the son of Irish immigrants who turned to the beauty industry during the Great Depression. He studied cosmetology, became a hairdresser and by the 1950s started teaching. Redding is credited with inventing the modern-day hair conditioner. He believed that hair was very much alive, not dead, and could be enhanced with the right treatments. He sought to create a product that used proteins, an integral component of our hair, to rebuild and repair damaged locks. Redding subsequently released the Jheri Redding Creme Rinse conditioner. As a businessman, he founded Redken Laboratories, and also Nexxus Products. The popularity of pH-balanced hair products is also attributed to Redding, as are shampoos and conditioners fortified with proteins.

The term pH is a figure that describes the level of acidity or basicity in an aqueous or liquid solution. Many of the products we use on our hair will increase its natural pH balance of 4.5 to 5.5, making our hair slightly acidic. The pH scale ranges from 0 to 14, with anything up to 6 being acidic. A pH of 7 is neutral (water) and 8 to 14 would be classified as alkaline.

By the late 70s, many of Redding's products were sold in salons across the States, including his Jheri curl products, although it was the African American entrepreneur Comer Cottrell who was responsible for making the curly perm more accessible. He created kits that men and women could buy in stores and apply themselves at home, making the curly perm much more affordable. Comer founded the Pro-Line Corporation in the 1970s, a Black haircare company based in Los Angeles, known for its bestselling product the Curly Kit. He pitched his company as 'A Black Manufacturer That Understands the Hair Care Needs of Black Consumers'.[1] The popularity of his products was clear for all to see, with many celebrities sporting and popularizing the look. This allowed him to export his products globally, reaching countries including Nigeria, Kenya, Trinidad and even Taiwan. Probably one of the most famous wearers of the Jheri curl in the 80s was Michael Jackson, who debuted the style on his 1982 album cover and video for the song 'Thriller'.

CASE STUDY

Short and curly

I have a client, a French actress, who keeps her hair short and neat on a regular basis and loves the look of curls. She doesn't have time to do natural sets (an alternative way to achieve a curly look), due to the demands of work and family. She came to the salon wanting a look that was curly but also easy to manage, a sort of get-up-and-go style that didn't take long to achieve, especially in the mornings. We both felt the longevity of a curly perm would be a good option, a more convenient way to achieve the sort of ease and glamour she needed. The new formulas for curly perms are drier and not as oily and greasy as the products from the 80s. I use small rods to create tiny, spiral-shaped curls all over her head and her daily maintenance includes the use of an activator and a moisturizer to maintain the curls. The actress visits the salon every four months. In between salon visits, I advise weekly mask treatments (as chemical treatments tend to dry out the hair) and, of course, a regular trim. Chemical treatments like the curly perm have advanced since they first came on the market. These days, they're not as dangerous, due to the use of better ingredients and the addition of more oils and conditioners as a way to further protect the hair from damage.

TIPS & TRICKS

Natural sets

Average styling time: 3 hours

Style duration: 1 to 2 weeks

Many clients come to the salon requesting more definition to their curls. But after the consultation, nine out of ten decide against a chemical treatment to achieve the look. The beauty of using tools such as rods, bendy rollers and drinking straws is that you can achieve a curly head of hair without chemicals. Natural sets are versatile as they work on natural, relaxed or transitioning hair and serve a variety of hair lengths. Rods, bendy rollers and drinking straws all come in different sizes.

Women with shorter hair tend to sport smaller, tighter curls while women with medium to longer lengths achieve more buoyant curls. The style can last anywhere from one to two weeks without having to shampoo, condition and apply products on a daily basis. The rods can be set on damp or dry hair, although the latter is recommended for kinkier textures to avoid extra shrinkage. Rods are good for tighter, S-shaped curls; bendy rollers are better for zigzag-shaped curls; drinking straws give more of a kinky coil. But this all depends on the hair type.

Tools you will need

- Rods, rollers or straws
- Tail comb to divide the hair into small sections
- A product to set the hair (what you decide to use depends on your hair type: kinky hair usually requires more of a hold, so a cream or gel works best, while a mousse or setting lotion would suit curlier hair textures)
- End papers (square-cut fibre papers) to gather the ends of the hair (the papers make the hair stay in one place when rolling the rods, rollers or straws)
- A mixture of oil, water and conditioner to spritz on after the set is complete (this helps to seal in moisture and gives it a nice sheen once hair is dry)

Step by step

1. Start at the nape of the neck and part a two-inch horizontal row using the tail comb. Then take a small section of hair within the row (about another two inches).
2. Depending on your hair type, apply the mousse, gel, cream or oil. Avoid saturating the hair. It's best to apply the products section by section to help the rods, rollers and straws stay in place for a solid curl.
3. Comb through and wrap an end paper at the tip of the hair.

4. Roll the section of hair around the rod, roller or straw until you reach the scalp. Use the attached band to secure or use a hairpin. If using bendy rollers, twist the roller onto itself to lock in place.

5. Repeat Steps 1 to 4 until you've completed the entire head.

6. Leave the hair to air-dry if doing the style at home. You can sleep with the bendy rollers overnight as they're made of foam. If you must use heat, due to time restrictions, sit under a hooded dryer for about thirty minutes. Allow the hair to cool for five minutes afterwards.

7. Ensure that the hair is completely dry before removing the rods, as hair that is still damp will not form correctly.

8. Separate the curls with your fingers a couple of times, depending on the desired look. You can also use an Afro Pik at the base of the hair to gently lift the curls for more volume. Use a lightweight finishing mist to help moisturize and define the curls and to hold the style in place.

Sleep with a silk or satin scarf or pillowcase at night. The best way to wrap a curly look is to put the scarf around the hairline, piling the curls on top of the head in a pineapple shape. Shower with a plastic cap to keep the curls dry.

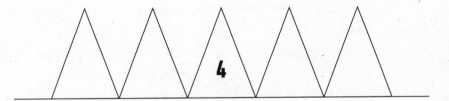

4

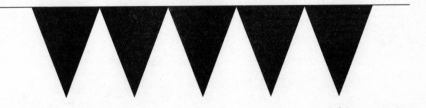

THE APPRENTICE

HAIR DISCRIMINATION PAST AND PRESENT

The experiences I had upon my return to England from Ghana have yet to become history. The policing of Black hairstyles continues to be a traumatic experience for young people in schools and for women in the workplace. Having worked within Afro haircare for over twenty years, I often come across clients working in the beauty or entertainment industries, where the freedom to express yourself is encouraged. Of course, over the years, I've also come across women who chemically straighten their hair or wear weaves in order to fit into a workplace. This is nothing new. But I was shocked to discover the number of online articles addressing cases of hair discrimination in the UK in both corporate settings and schools, where cultural integration has yet to take place. Many of these institutions seem to be fearful or ignorant of styles indigenous to our race, ethnicity and culture. They also seem to maintain and uphold outdated ideas of Eurocentric beauty, conscious and unconscious baggage, perpetuated from as far back as the seventeenth century, as highlighted in previous chapters.

British sociology academics Dr Remi Joseph-Salisbury and Dr Laura Connelly draw connections between the treatment of the enslaved by slavemasters (through the control and domination of hair) and how this same use of power is played out in many of our cultural institutions today. Enslaved people were forced to shave their heads, as mentioned in Chapter 1, but there were also examples of masters' wives who, out of jealousy and due to philandering husbands, cut off the hair of Black female house slaves as a means of punishment and control.

There have been many high-profile cases across the UK and US, in particular, that have dominated the press over the past several years regarding Black hair and dress codes in the workplace and within schools. Many of the policies that govern our key institutions were simply not written by a sufficiently diverse group of people, never mind considerations being made for race, culture and ethnicity.

Women and children are penalized the most for hairstyles that are considered improper, with words such as 'extreme' and 'unusual' often used to describe Black hair within these institutions. In 2016, the BBC published an article online about the stigma of Afro hair in London workplaces. A woman named Leila explained to the journalist that her employer asked her repeatedly to disguise her Afro hair by wearing a weave. Leila goes on to say that many of her co-workers made her feel as if wearing her hair naturally was 'unprofessional' for the workplace. She also had this to say about wearing one of her protective styles: 'A few years ago I had my hair styled in cornrows and I was asked quite blatantly by my boss how long it would be before my hair was back to "normal".[1] Leila eventually opted to wear a weave to avoid further tensions and future problems.

In America, high-profile examples of discrimination against cornrows came to light after a landmark case in 1981, when an American Airlines ticket agent in the US was fired for wearing the style. She took her claim to court but the judge ruled against her, stating the style had nothing to do with her heritage. Instead, the judge claimed that the style was influenced by the white actress Bo Derek. In 2014, the United States Army updated their grooming and appearance policy to say that staff were not allowed to wear cornrows or dreadlocks, braids or twists, although the language they used excluded references to race.[2] Yet, in 2017, they overruled their policy to allow dreadlocks.

The way a woman of colour, and in particular a Black woman, decides to wear her hair often determines whether she'll be accepted for a job or even fired for not complying with unspoken dress code policies. The wearing of weaves or choosing to chemically straighten the hair allows many Black women in the workplace to fit in with white colleagues. These hairstyles prevent unwanted attention or insensitive comments, but sometimes have a negative psychological impact.

The implication is that the system dictates the way we should look and takes away our right to express who we naturally are. Although most policies do not explicitly state that Afros or certain protective styles aren't allowed in the workplace, it's obvious from Leila's example and many others that there are unwritten ideologies in place that are enforced and practised every day. Speaking up often has adverse implications within institutions that don't care to understand (or celebrate) the differences that exist between cultures, and many women are forced to carry and live with feelings of shame or inferiority. It takes a lot of bravery to insist upon our natural textures and hairstyles being allowed in these spaces, but sometimes it's worth speaking up.

This was demonstrated by the 2017 Chikayzea Flanders case when a twelve-year-old Black boy turned up to his first day of school only to be told that his dreadlocks were against school policy. He was given the ultimatum of cutting them off, otherwise he would face suspension, and until that point, he would be taught in isolation. His mother eventually pulled him out of school. She also took legal action against the London primary for discriminating against the family's Rastafarian religion, as dreadlocks are an integral part of their belief system. Dr Remi Joseph-Salisbury and Dr Laura Connelly also draw parallels between the idea of dreadlocks being 'messy' and 'unkempt' and the belief that those who wear the style must be lacking in discipline or academic rigour. It's no mistake that Black hair within this Eurocentric viewpoint is consistently seen as 'distracting' or 'too expressive', and many examples of a need to exert correctness continually play out. A year later, in the US, a video went viral of a young boy at a wrestling match who was told by a referee to either cut off his dreadlocks, there and then, or forfeit the match along with his entire team. The video then shows the boy in tears as his locs are cut by a stranger.

Journalist Micha Frazer-Carroll published an article in the *Huffington Post* about hair discrimination in which she describes her sister's experience at the age of nine at a North London primary school. One day she showed up to school wearing braids with beads at the end and was told to remove both the braids and the beads as they were 'inappropriate'. 'I remember the way it made me feel so clearly, like by having braids I had done something wrong – and subconsciously I internalized the idea that something about my Blackness was inherently bad,' she says.[3] What many schools and teachers fail to realize is that these styles are expressions of our heritage and cultures. They date back to our ancestors and serve as important protective styles that help maintain the health and integrity of our hair. Although steps are being taken, especially in New York, to ban hair-based discrimination, much work still needs to be done around the education of Black hair in the workplace and in schools.

SPLINTERS: AN EDUCATION IN BLACK HAIRCARE

When I reflect on the fact that my career has centred around the celebration of Black hair and the wealth of styles afforded to us, I can't help but feel blessed. Although I lost my mum in such a tragic way, it led me to discover a lifelong passion. When a careers officer visited my school a couple of years after Mum died, I realized that I wanted to pursue hairdressing as a professional career, as it had given me solace during a turbulent time and was something I truly wanted to master.

The officer recommended a work-based training course called the Youth Training Scheme (YTS), designed for school leavers aged sixteen and seventeen. I was offered a chance to work at premier salons such as Vidal Sassoon, Sanrizz or Roots. But there was an upscale Afro hair salon in Mayfair called Splinters that sounded just right, so the officer scheduled a meeting with the founder, Winston Isaacs. Alongside four days at the salon, I'd also spend one day a week at the London College of Fashion, the most happening place to study in 1986 if you were interested in the arts and anything creative. It wasn't uncommon to see some of the world's best fashion designers, like Stella McCartney and Alexander McQueen, working away in the library or eating in the dining halls. The training at college instilled the science and theory of hairdressing, but the education I received at Splinters would be hands-on.

The day of my interview, I came out of Oxford Street tube station and walked along Regent Street. I'd never been to that part of London in my life, so just seeing the posh shops and the bright lights, the hustling and bustling, felt very different from the world I was living in. I showed up to the salon on Maddox Street an hour early and felt as if I were walking into a five-star hotel. What I didn't know at the time was that Splinters had the reputation of a destination salon. Celebrities from all over the world came on their private jets to get their hair done or had chauffeurs waiting for them outside. Big-time entertainers like Diana Ross and Janet Jackson had all visited the space. It was the only professional Black hair salon bang in the West End, known for its excellence and expertise. Splinters was composed of three floors, with a reception area and cloakroom on the ground floor, a hair academy at the back, and the salon spreading over two floors, with styling on the upper floors and shampooing, colouring and chemical services in the basement. The atmosphere was lively, full of young Black stylists who all looked very happy. There was never a day when there wasn't music playing and someone dancing, not to mention the over-the-top clients who greeted you with phrases like, 'Hello, dahling!' Walking into Splinters felt like progress; I finally felt on my way after the passing of my mum only a few years earlier. When I met Winston for my interview, we got on very well. I was astonished by how tall he was, the way he carried himself, and how he looked down at me from his glasses. Winston spoke well, smelled nice and looked smart. He could be strict but very charming. He was a father figure to many of us and taught by example.

He opened Splinters promptly at 9 a.m. and all employees had to be at work fifteen minutes before. If anyone showed up even five minutes after that, he would tell them off. We weren't allowed to chew gum and were always expected to show up groomed, with our hygiene, appearance and posture in check. 'Whatever problems you've got,' he'd say, 'leave them outside the door. You're here for work.' But, of course, there were always exceptions to the rule. There were many, many times I felt sad about what had happened with Mum. He'd sit me down for a chat and give me a hug, so it wasn't always business as usual. Winston cared about us and our futures. He showed us how to read hair properly and impressed on us the dangers of cutting corners.

During our first and second years, we shadowed stylists and watched their every move. We brought them tea and lunch, announced their clients and handed them their rollers, and in our third year we became junior stylists. Our training was very systematic, and we moved from one stage to the next when Winston felt we were ready. If you were shampooing, you shampooed until you were the best shampooist. If you were colouring, you coloured until you were the best colourist. The same applied when learning to provide specialist services like curly perms, which were all the rage. My hands looked like prunes by the end of the day because of the constant neutralizing. If you happened to do a particularly good neutralizer, your stylist would take note and praise you at the weekly meeting, making you the star of the week.

Besides the curly perm, women often emulated popular American R&B and hip hop groups like Shalamar, Total Contrast, Sinitta, and Cedella and Ziggy Marley. So chemical treatments, in general, were in demand along with bouncy blow-dries. During our model nights, we showed off what we'd learned during the week, whether it was something as simple as a good blow-dry or setting and wrapping. If Winston felt you were progressing quickly, he'd move you to the next stage. Our training was slow and steady – not like these days, when anyone can be a stylist on YouTube or Instagram after 1,000 likes. Things were different, back then. Kids were eager to learn without the rush or adrenaline of trying to make big bucks too quickly.

We earned very little in those days, about £27 a week, but we relied heavily on tips. We could make more than our wages in a day, but then again, everything was a lot cheaper in the 80s, and most of us lived at home or in paid-for accommodation.

Splinters became my home away from home. A place where I felt happy and free. It was a breath of fresh air being around my own culture and no longer being bullied because I came from Ghana or had dark skin. School felt so mundane to me, the same old, repetitive thing. At Splinters, I could participate in the transformation of others, and that was such a satisfying experience. It almost felt like therapy, and it took a lot of my own pain and suffering away. At school, I felt so mixed up all the time and singled out, but at Splinters we all had a common interest: Afro hair. Students came from all over London, from Peckham to Tottenham, to train – and we all seemed to have similar experiences of school. Not everyone who studied at Splinters succeeded in the hair industry; many went on to do other things like nursing or further education. But there are those of us who persevered – like Junior Green, Errol Douglas, Johnnie Sarpong and Desmond Murray – and turned our studying into a career.

The beauty of our education stemmed from the diversity of our days. One day, we'd all make a trip to Kensington Town Hall for an Afro Hair and Beauty show, where big brands like Dark and Lovely, Sta-Sof-Fro, Ultra Sheen, TCB and Optimum would come and do demos of their products (all chemically based at the time, as clients in those days were obsessed with curly perms or relaxers). Another day, we might be off to a show on behalf of a client who'd given us tickets to see her husband's play. I remember *Black Heroes in the Hall of Fame*, a showcase of prominent Black figures from the seventeenth to nineteenth centuries. I'd never heard of these figures in my history books, so going to the show enriched and empowered me as a seventeen-year-old Black girl at the time. My education at Splinters and under Winston's tutelage made me feel limitless. The experience became a part of my DNA. It built and shaped me, and somehow followed me until everything slowly but surely came together.

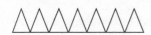

My education at Splinters and under Winston's tutelage made me feel limitless. The experience became a part of my DNA. It built and shaped me, and somehow followed me until everything slowly but surely came together.

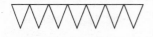

TIPS & TRICKS

How to get the most out of your salon consultation

One of the best things to do before heading to the salon is to do your research and book in a consultation with a stylist. If you're looking for a cheaper alternative to a salon visit, especially for children's services or a simple cut, a junior stylist is a great option. They are recently qualified and new to the profession, therefore commanding a lower fee. They are usually also working towards their respective accredited qualification. Junior stylists help senior stylists with daily tasks such as shampooing, mixing colour, meeting and greeting clients, and keeping the salon tidy.

A fully fledged stylist, on the other hand, works independently. They've already gained their qualifications and experience and will perform a range of tasks like cutting and hair colouring. Lastly, senior stylists have the skills to deliver the highest quality of service and, as a result, command a much higher fee for their time. They train and mentor junior stylists and can take on other titles, such as creative or artistic director. Their experience behind the chair is vast, so you should book in with a senior stylist if you're looking for advanced cutting, styling and colouring services.

When speaking with your chosen stylist, be as direct as possible. Discuss what you want to change, your hair routine, what you feel is possible and not possible. Tell your stylist if you're low maintenance so that they can create a cut or style that's easy to manage. A stylist will suggest what they think will look best on you, depending on your face shape, hair type and lifestyle. Bring in an inspirational picture of a style or colour that you want to emulate. A good stylist, whether they're junior or senior, will spend a good amount of time making sure they're on the same page as the client. They will explain shapes and tones and manageability.

TAKING CARE OF BUSINESS

Although Splinters saved my career, other parts of my life were still unstable. A friend at Splinters gave me some advice regarding an organization called the Ujima Housing Association, which, back then, offered accommodation for under-privileged women of Afro-Caribbean descent lacking family support. After my meeting, within a fortnight, I was offered a temporary room in a hostel belonging to GAP House (the Girls Alone Project) shared with nine other girls. I came home from work one evening and told my dad I was leaving home. Once I'd made up my mind, the decision was final. The next day he drove me to Oakley Square in Mornington Crescent. I finally got the freedom I was craving, and felt empowered by it. Now I could take a short bus ride to work and come and go as I pleased. But the allure of living alone soon lost its appeal when one morning, around 4 a.m., I woke to a group of boys in my basement bedroom. They were high on drugs and in the middle of stealing everything I owned. I still thank God that I went untouched, but I found it very hard to relax in my own space after that.

Six months later, GAP House offered me my own flat and I moved into 13b Wren Street, in King's Cross. Although I was grateful to finally have my own place, I still felt very lonely. Sometimes I'd bring my siblings to the flat, but I didn't always have the energy after work, and they weren't old enough to ride the bus on their own. By this time, I'd graduated from Splinters and began working with a stylist who opened up her own salon in Battersea. She felt like a mum to me and invited me over for home-cooked meals after work with some of her other friends. Although I was grateful for the company, I couldn't always relate to the older women and still felt very lost.

The day my eldest sister invited me to a christening changed my life forever. I was twenty years old at the time and quite the party girl. If you lived on your own, with no parents telling you what to do, you literally did what you liked. I loved hip hop and house music raves like Sunrise and Biology and often hung out with a group of friends who knew which DJs could get us on the list for all the best parties in town. There were times when we weren't so lucky and had to wait by the radio just to hear where the venue would be for the night. I remember going out from Saturday to Monday morning, partying in fields in towns like

Dunstable, with DJs like Grooverider spinning tunes. One of my favourite London venues at the time was the Arches in Vauxhall. It's not the same any more, but every artist you could think of would come over from America to play a gig there. Subterania in Notting Hill was another happening place where artists like Lil' Kim and Foxy Brown came to play. My connections in the hair world often invited me to Def Jam parties and, in those days, I met quite a few music managers, one of whom used to look after Warren G.

At the christening, I was introduced to a mysterious man, someone completely different from what I was used to. I fancied hip hop artists like Method Man and Big Daddy Kane (who I'd seen three times at Brixton Academy between the ages of seventeen and nineteen), and I was a little nervous to meet this man who was calm and correct, quiet and respectful. He had a good job and seemed very mature, and in time he became my husband, but not before I fell pregnant with my first child at twenty-two. My life changed in that moment forever. It sobered me. It made me get serious, as I had new responsibilities. The bond I shared with my son was unlike anything I'd ever felt. Now, I no longer needed to cook only for me. Now, I had a family, people to love and support. But having a child meant that I needed to find better accommodation. I decided to go to my local MP's surgery, where I often went to seek advice, and I spoke to Frank Dobson, the Labour MP at the time, who, out of kindness and a stroke of luck, wrote a letter to the Camden Housing

Association. Shortly after that, they relocated me to Notting Hill, to the beautiful flat I live in today. It wasn't until all of these pieces came together that I started to think about taking hair more seriously.

HAIRSTYLES THROUGH THE AGES

Relaxers and chemical treatments

Relaxers became a very popular and reliable way for Black women to straighten their hair for a longer period of time. Scientists began researching more efficient ways to straighten hair, and by the mid-1950s an active ingredient was found that could break the disulphide bonds of the hair – sodium hydroxide, often called lye in the States or caustic soda in the UK. The compound was blended into creams and applied to new growth on Afro hair or all over the head. The chemical treatment left hair in a smooth state, somewhere between six to eight weeks before new growth reappeared. The African American businessman George E. Johnson of Johnson Products introduced a range of relaxers and cream-press permanents containing lye, which he sold in stores so that men and women could apply them at home. Men were also finding ways to straighten their hair, using a method called the 'conk', in which they blended together lye and household items such as eggs. Although home kits were widely available, it was often advised to have the treatment done by a professional in a salon as the sodium hydroxide in the cream could burn the scalp if left on for too long.

During the early days, bases or protective creams were used around the scalp and hairline to protect the sensitive areas from the alkaline nature of sodium hydroxide. Most relaxers have a pH of 11 or 12 but some can be as low as 10 or as high as 14, making them extremely alkaline. Years later, the use of a base was no longer needed as formulas were enhanced to be safer, and they included ingredients that aided in the conditioning of the scalp. I still advise using a base. Sodium hydroxide was seen as an expedient way to straighten the hair; the greater the concentration of the chemical, the less time the relaxer needed to stay on the hair. Depending on the hair type, a scale of relaxer strengths was created, from mild to regular to super. Women and men with Type 4C hair would typically use the super strength, for example, and those with colour-treated hair would use a mild strength, because of the already sensitive nature of the hair.

Relaxers are not as popular as they used to be some twenty years ago, most likely due to their toxicity and subsequent long-term damage. In the early 90s and 2000s, nine out of ten women who rang the salon on Portobello Road were calling to get a relaxer or a weave, with the latter now being extremely popular due to the ability to wear one's natural hair underneath.

Precautions should be taken when applying relaxers. In general, it's typical for clients to wait eight to twelve weeks before undertaking another treatment after new growth has appeared. The chemical treatment should not be applied to hair that's just come out of a protective style, such as braiding or cornrowing, due to the sensitive nature of the scalp. Relaxers should also never be applied to scalps that have scratches, cuts or abrasions. I would advise waiting about a week or two and would recommend a deep conditioning treatment beforehand.

TIPS & TRICKS

Tex-laxing

Average styling time: 15 minutes

Style duration: 10 to 12 weeks

Tex-laxing is a good option for those wanting to ease themselves off relaxers or those who are not completely comfortable with wearing their hair naturally, due to work pressures or a lack of knowledge about how to care for and maintain Afro hair. The process involves using relaxer treatments to under-process the hair. The chemical treatment is left on for a shorter period of time, instead of what's prescribed on the kit, which is usually about fifteen minutes plus. Hair is left textured but not completely straight and allows clients with Afro hair to achieve a softer, straighter look. Tex-laxing also helps to release your natural curl pattern, adding a lot more sheen. You can do this at home, although I always recommend that chemical services be done by a professional in a reputable salon. There's always the risk of leaving the relaxer on for too long, or additional breakage between differing textures of hair.

Tools you will need

- Mild to normal relaxer with applicator comb or brush
- Gloves
- Barrier cream or scalp protector
- Conditioner or oil

Step by step

1. Protect the scalp and hair by using a barrier cream or scalp protector. This slows down the relaxing process.
2. Apply a mild to normal relaxer, depending on your curl pattern. I recommend that if you try this method at home, you add conditioner or oil to the relaxer mix to dilute the formula adequately.
3. Do not smooth or comb through to the ends. Keep on for a maximum of fifteen minutes.
4. Wash out the chemical treatment thoroughly with shampoo and conditioner, and style as normal.

COLOURING YOUR HAIR

Splinters gave me an excuse to constantly have a new do, as stylists needed models to show off a new look. One day, a stylist cut my hair into a graduated bob, then dyed the back of my shaved head a bright orange. When I returned home to Edmonton that day, my father exclaimed, 'What's wrong with you? Have you seen the back of your head? It looks like someone set it on fire!' Despite what my father thought, I felt cool. No one in the neighbourhood had a cut and colour as good as mine. When strangers stopped me on the street to ask where I got my hair done, I'd proudly say, 'Splinters.'

Hair colouring is an excellent way to change your everyday appearance. There are so many colours out there, these days, and so many different ways to apply them, from temporary colours to semi-permanents and permanents. It's common practice for both men and women to use colouring as a means of disguising grey hairs. Others colour their hair to spruce up their look, whether they want something bold and funky or traditional yet different to their normal colour.

Hair dyes are usually made from chemical substances, although henna, a natural hair colourant made from the leaves of the henna tree, is still used today in India, the Middle East and North Africa to temporarily dye the hair a reddish brown. Henna goes back as far as the Ancient Egyptians, who used a variety of plants and the blood of animals to dye the hair. According to Victoria Sherrow, the invention of hair dye as a chemical treatment appeared around the 1900s when a French chemist named Eugene Schueller used paraphenylenediamine, a chemical discovered in 1863 and originally used to dye textiles, to create his own products. He would later go on to name his company L'Oréal after several name changes and reinventions.

Hair dye can be bought in stores as a kit or applied by a professional in a salon. Temporary colours come in the form of mousses, rinses or gels, sprays and paints, and usually wash out after one shampoo. Semi-permanents provide an additional layer of vibrant colour to the hair and only darken your strands as they don't contain ingredients such as peroxide, ammonia or alcohol. They offer the chance to change your colour more frequently without the commitment of a permanent. The colour rests on the hair shaft only, so the effect is temporary and washes out over a period of time – usually within several weeks to a couple of months, or less than a dozen washes. Semi-permanents are usually applied after hair has been shampooed and dried, making the hair more accepting of the colour. Shampooing opens up the cuticle and removes sebum, which acts as a barrier to the colour. Permanents, on the other hand, need sebum to act as a lubricant before the colour is applied, otherwise the colour would irritate the scalp, and therefore it's advised that hair is unwashed before application. A moisturizing conditioner will usually be applied to Afro hair before a permanent, for the same protective results. If considering colouring grey hairs, a permanent is always best as semi-permanents cannot completely dye them. The cortex is completely saturated by colour during a permanent. The colour of your natural hair is altered, either lightened or darkened by several shades, because of the ammonia or peroxide, which means that the colour cannot be washed out and has a longer-lasting effect. Permanent colours need to grow out or be bleached, if dyed again.

Be mindful with colouring – a recent study in the US has found a strong correlation between the use of permanent colour among African American women and cancer, which they estimate as increasing risk by approximately 45 per cent.[4] The study suggested a link between the way that the dye is applied on Black women's hair and a difference in hair texture as a potential reason.

CASE STUDY

Colour it in

A fashion designer/stylist was in desperate need of a new colour and style after concealing her hair under hats and scarves for weeks. Her hair was already in good condition, which is helpful when considering a colour treatment, as hair that's damaged won't take to a colour treatment (and it will further destroy the strands). I thought a light blonde orange-red would suit her complexion, taking the outgrown blonde to a more vibrant shade while enhancing her cheekbones. We decided to cut the sides and back to give her a more dramatic look and to opt for china bumps, a part-threaded, part-Bantu knot hairstyle. Before applying any sort of colour it's important to stabilize the colour and give hair extra protection, so I treated the client's hair with a revitalizing oil.

I coloured the hair with a blonde tint and left it on to develop for thirty minutes, to lift the hair up three shades. ('Lifting' simply means that the hair is being stripped of some of its natural colour while the dye is deposited into the strands.) The colour was then thoroughly rinsed out and a light blonde orange-red colourant applied, which I left on for a further twenty minutes. After a rinse off and towel dry, I used an oil restorative hair mask and combed it through. Masks help to hydrate and repair colour-treated hair and this one was rich in argan oil and proteins, which assist in fortifying and restructuring the hair as well as providing shine and manageability. Hair was cut very low at the sides and back using clippers to provide more definition. An essential oil was then applied and combed through with a wide toothcomb to straighten out any kinky curls.

Lastly, I divided the hair into thirteen sections. Using half a metre of black thread in my right hand, I held each section of hair at the scalp between my left thumb and forefinger. After anchoring the end of the thread by twisting it around the hair at the scalp a few times, I knotted the thread to avoid unravelling. I repeated the entire process with each of the sections until the entire head was threaded.

Balayage technique

Balayage is a French word meaning to paint or sweep and is a bespoke hand-painted highlighting technique that can work on a variety of hair lengths and types. If you're looking for a less dramatic makeover, highlights are a good way to enhance your colour without transforming your entire head of hair. Highlights involve dyeing pieces of hair a lighter colour than the base colour of your hair. The Balayage method highlights the hair in more natural and subtle ways, compared to the foil highlights of the past, which leave the hair looking stripy. The colour is applied on the surface of the hair, working from the roots downwards, with a heavier and more saturated application towards the mid-length and ends, depending on the desired effect. The Balayage technique targets smaller, more strategic pieces of hair decided upon by the stylist and is a great way to accentuate a good haircut as well as the natural tones found in an individual's skin and hair. Unlike foil highlights, which require more maintenance and salon visits, the Balayage technique grows out or fades more naturally. It's also a faster process than foil highlights but is best left to a professional.

CASE STUDY

Highlighted

I had a student visit the salon once who found it really difficult to style her curly hair. She wanted a nice cut but also a change of colour. I suggested we restyle her hair by cutting it into layers to create more volume. I felt the Balayage technique would suit the new cut and recommended incorporating terracotta tones through the mid-length and ends of the hair. It's important to stabilize the colour and to give the hair extra protection, so I pre-treated the hair with a shea butter and essential oil masque. I then bleached her hair, leaving the dye on for twenty minutes, so the hair lifted up two levels. The bleach was then rinsed off and the hair treated with a moisturizing shampoo. A semi-permanent orange-red tone was applied to the mid-length and ends for twenty-five minutes. After rinsing the colour off thoroughly, I conditioned the hair with a moisturizing shea butter conditioner.

Last but not least, the client's hair was cut into layers before applying a moisturizing cream and then stretching and dividing the hair into eight sections for blow-drying. It's useful to comb out and twist each section of hair loosely, to keep it separated. This makes blow-drying much easier. The roots were dried to stretch out the curls and the style finished off with more moisturizing cream before stretching and finger-combing into shape.

TIPS & TRICKS

Protecting and preserving your colour

Here are some simple tips to ensure you make the most of your new look.

- Use gentle moisturizing shampoos and conditioners (go to 'Reading the small print' on page 216 to find out more about ingredients best avoided).
- Visit the salon for follow-up moisturizing and protein treatments.
- Keep hair trimmed regularly.
- Avoid sun and chlorine, as both will dry out the hair and possibly change its colour. The sun also damages colour-treated hair. Protect it from UVA using moisturizing hair products containing sunscreen.

- The less you manipulate your hair with heated appliances, the better. This includes hairdryers, flat irons, curling irons, etc. Heat will add stress to hair that has been weakened by the chemical process.
- If you're looking for a more permanent colour, it's important to have your hair touched up at least every four to six weeks to maintain the consistency of the new shade.
- If opting for a semi-permanent, it will last longer when applied after the conditioning treatment.
- Avoid products with petroleum (such as Vaseline) as these will cause unnecessary build-up.
- Avoid products with alcohol as these will strip the hair of natural oils.

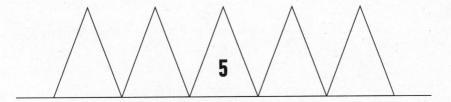

5

GOING INTO BUSINESS

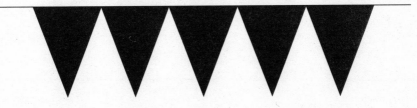

NOTTING HILL AND THE CARIBBEAN COMMUNITY

In June of 1948, a ship called the SS *Windrush* left Kingston, Jamaica for London. Although it was advertised as only having room for about 300 passengers to board, it was filled to the brim with an estimated 500 occupants including ex-servicemen, tradesmen and, equally, stowaways. Black servicemen from the Caribbean were returning to Britain in droves in search of economic prosperity and, more importantly, to play a vital role in the post-war reconstruction of Britain. They had lived in and served the country and were eager to return to the land of milk and honey. Tickets for travel came to £28.10,[1] and long queues formed as people were eager for employment and a better way of life. The author Edward Scobie writes that the British Government boasted of more work for its citizens. But in the case of Black immigrants to the UK, this meant menial jobs such as street cleaners, construction site labourers or laundry maids, and eventually, slightly more lucrative jobs such as bus drivers and railway conductors. Between 1949 and 1962, immigrants from the Caribbean were coming in large numbers to live and work, until the passing of the Commonwealth Immigrants Act, which made it considerably harder for Black migrants to come to the UK.

Neighbourhoods across London were establishing more of a Caribbean flavour as men and women migrated to specific boroughs to join their family and friends. Bustling Jamaican communities could be found in Clapham and Brixton, with an especially high proportion of Trinidadians setting up shop in Notting Hill. Black immigrants found it difficult to rent from white landlords due to racism, with advertisements stating 'no blacks' or 'no coloureds'. Landlords found that if they kept Black tenants, they could no longer rent to white people, who didn't want to live in close proximity. They also found that the values of their properties would depreciate. Landlords who rented to Blacks often doubled or tripled the rent for uninhabitable places to make up for losses, and this spurred many Caribbean families to save money to buy a place of their own. Immigrants were often accused of having a lifestyle not in keeping with British sensibilities, from the fragrant food to the vibrant parties.

One of the most famous slum landlords around Notting Hill at the time was a man named Peter Rachman, a Polish immigrant and property developer whose criminal acts and lavish lifestyle have taken on mythic proportions. He was known to rent to those looked down upon by society, such as West Indians, just as long as he made a profit, and he was both vilified and respected in equal measure. In an article on 'Rachmanism', writer Caryl Phillips states that Rachman paid Caribbean lodgers to play loud music day and night as a way to drive white tenants out of his properties so he could inflate the price of his flats. He also 'hired black hoodlums to intimidate white tenants, or, conversely, white hoodlums to harass black tenants; and if these tactics failed, Rachman would employ thugs with Alsatian dogs to wrench doors off their hinges, remove roof tiles, and rip up floorboards in order to terrify those he wished to evict.'[2]

The areas that many Caribbeans had come to call home became increasingly dangerous as it became sport for white teenage boys and men, especially Teddy boys, to run riot and target the local Black populations. Homes and shops were vandalized, and racist slogans put up, and all of the hate gave rise to the Notting Hill race riots of August and September 1958. By the mid-1960s and 70s Notting Hill began to change, with a sense of the Caribbean community flowering, grounded in resilience. The annual Notting Hill Carnival was the vision of Tobagan Claudia Jones, a former member of the Communist Party in the US. She pioneered a Mardi Gras-style carnival in 1959, bringing together locals, associations, councils and schools, which contributed to the carnival through grants, loans and participation on the day.

The neighbourhood saw the rise of new inhabitants, from pop stars and musicians to radicals and liberals, to artists and the wealthy. It came to be known as (and still is) Kensington's 'artsy little brother'. The carnival became a melting pot of people coming together to forge a new identity and politics, and everyone wanted a piece of the celebration, which came to represent West Indian history, culture and presence in the UK. But carnival was not without tension between participants and police, and the carnival of 1976, among others, grew out of control. Alongside the joy and momentary freedom of expression came detractors, those who felt the celebration to be another example of Black waywardness and criminality, a view which is sadly still published in papers today.

Despite the naysayers, my experience of carnival has always been memorable and fun. I still remember my first time, at seventeen years old. The lot of us who worked at Splinters were invited to ride a float sponsored by the American haircare brand Dark and Lovely. We were glowing that day, feeling like celebrities, with friends and family waving and calling out our names. Even then, I knew how special the borough was, with its unique blend of creativity and culture. I never dreamed (at the time) that I would live there, let alone have my very own salon.

SALON HOPPING

After my stroke of luck with Frank Dobson, Labour MP, my husband and I moved to Notting Hill in 1993, when I was twenty-two with a six-month-old baby in tow. I fell in love with my new home and neighbourhood with its mixture of families, parks and markets, not to mention Notting Hill Carnival every year! I was lucky to have family who lived within walking distance who could help with babysitting whenever my husband and I went to work. The area was a breath of fresh air after the chopping and changing of the last few years, living alone, and trying to make ends meet without help or community. It was as soon as I moved to Notting Hill that my life started making more sense.

After my apprenticeship at Splinters I moved on to working at Lapaz in Notting Hill and Camden and at Xtension Masters. This was the mid-90s when weaves were blowing up and it was all about having a beautiful mane of long, flowing hair. I remember ringing up Xtension Masters after seeing an ad in *Black Hair* magazine, and I took my son along to the interview in his pram. I will never forget meeting the owner, Tai Arogundade, who asked me early on what I wanted to do in five years' time. I told her I wanted to run my own business, and when that eventually happened, she was the first person to ring me and say, 'You did it!' Tai must've been one of my first role models as she was a woman in her late twenties, full of tenacity and drive, with a young son also in her care. She was running a salon, writing for *Sophisticate's Black Hair Styles*, and it was almost like I was seeing myself in about ten years' time.

Xtension Masters was a great place to work because it was all about extensions – and doing it well. Tai was brilliant at executing our timelines, and we managed clients three times a day (9 a.m., 1 p.m. and 3 p.m.) with the stylists leaving the salon at 6.30 p.m. sharp. Tai wanted people to respect her time and to be on time, so we all completed our weaves in about two and a half hours tops. Although I enjoyed my time at Xtension Masters, I yearned to use the other skills I'd learned at Splinters. I could cut and relax hair, and I could do a good blow-dry and colour, so eventually I moved on.

Next came Terry Jacques, a salon in South London, specializing in good professional Afro hair. The salon was based in Clapham, and every morning I found myself rushing to get my son ready for nursery and then rushing to get down south. Although I worked at the salon three or four days a week, I knew I wanted to spend more time at home with my son and so I started to pursue freelancing. Even whilst working at both salons, I continued to see clients in my home or theirs, and after about eight months at Terry Jacques, I decided to pursue working for myself.

I walked around the Notting Hill area, looking for a chair to rent. Surprisingly, I found a European salon in Westbourne Park Road called 10500. I asked if I could rent a chair to do Afro hair and they said yes. The environment was different to what I was used to, but I enjoyed the quirky stylists. I met one of my oldest friends at 10500; she is a mixed-race Swedish woman whose mother used to fly her over from Stockholm to get her hair done. Way back in 1996, her mother had found me by coincidence. One day she'd booked into a salon down the road when a fight near the premises broke out and someone was unfortunately shot. The whole area was cordoned off, when she met a stranger near Portobello Road who told her about a woman downstairs at 10500 who specialized in curly hair textures. She began bringing her daughter in to see me. In those days, chemical treatments were big. I relaxed her daughter's hair because she was obsessed with Beyoncé from her

Destiny's Child days and desired her locks long and straight. It's funny, that encounter tells you so much about the area I've come to call home, then and now: one of diversity.

Having a chair really helped me to manage my time and money but it also opened my eyes to what having a salon could be like. As my clientele grew at 10500, and as the price for my chair skyrocketed, I knew it was time to move on and find something more suitable to my needs.

At that moment, I wasn't exactly sure what the next move would be. I'd amassed a sizeable group of customers, some of whom I'd been styling since my days at Terry Jacques. On the one hand, I thought I could rent a seat elsewhere, but on the other, I knew it would be difficult to find something in West London that would allow me to tend to my clients but, equally, have the flexibility to be close to family. In the end, my own principles led me to the understanding that opening a salon would be the only way to go.

But where to start? I had experience being self-employed through renting my own seat, but this truly felt like another world. I didn't know the ins and outs of what was involved with starting a business, I wasn't even sure how to go about it and if I needed to register a name! What I did know was the power of my craft – and with that, I knew I could make it a success.

The best kind of innovation comes when utilizing the resources around you. For me, that came with discovering The Prince's Trust. I engaged with the organization with an open mind, and left with a grant that provided the capital to allow me to open the salon. That was pivotal, but what has proved to be of the most importance was the exposure it gave me to the world of business. I got a mentor, I learned how to write a business plan and, as a result, I was able to really drill down into why I wanted to do this. It's always downplayed, but having people you don't really know buy into your ideas, coupled with your own self-belief, is transformational. The drive was always there, but other people put the battery in my back to get there even faster, and for that I am forever grateful and supportive.

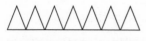

The best kind of innovation comes when utilizing the resources around you.

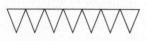

I worked from home to save money and, later, decided to get advice from the Portobello Business Centre, where they spoke to me about The Prince's Trust, a youth charity that helps young people get jobs, education and training. My mentor helped me secure a grant to start my own business, and this felt right, as I'd created solid foundations by this time with a steady flow of regular clients. I have recently become an ambassador for The Prince's Trust, working with young adults across London, instilling the same entrepreneurial values that the organization helped me refine all those years ago. I opened my first salon in 1999, at twenty-nine years old, in a studio space at the Imex Business Centre in Kilburn Park Road. I called it the Hair Lounge, from my days working from home where my sitting room became the waiting place for clients. The room became transformed into a space where women from all walks of life came together to share, grow and learn, and I wanted to recreate this same vibe in my very first salon. But moving from home to the business centre was a risky thing to do, as I didn't have a shop front. The centre housed plenty of businesses and workspaces, but future clients were unable to see me from the outside. I could sit in my studio twiddling my thumbs with all four of my empty chairs or I could be proactive, so I took out a small advert in *Black Beauty & Hair* magazine. I also managed to attract clients through word of mouth as parents from my son's school wanted to check out what I did, and from there they would bring friends, and friends of friends.

The business centre was a bustling place, full of creatives and entrepreneurs. One of my neighbours had a space where he made and sold custom belts, and on the other side of me, surprisingly, was a small church. One of the units upstairs sold home furnishings, and another belonged to UNICEF. Eventually, my time at the business centre came to an end. It was an all-round enriching experience that exposed me to the peaks and troughs of running a business. I learned it was always better to take risks and make mistakes than avoid them altogether. My experience up until then really highlighted that with business it's always better to crawl before you walk, and walk before you run. Needless to say, I was always plotting how I could get closer to realizing my dreams. In 2003, I felt it was time to embark on yet another journey. I wanted to be closer to home, especially now with my second child. My ultimate dream was to have a shop on Portobello Road, but I knew there were things standing in my way, such as gentrification, affordability and prejudice. The area had greatly changed in the last twenty years, with the influx of wealth and cult films like *Notting Hill*. What was once a bastion for Black business and entrepreneurship had somewhat ceased to exist, and I knew that the odds would be stacked against me as a Black woman trying to get a shop on Portobello Road.

The Hair Lounge (Portobello Road)

It took some time to find the perfect salon – and, believe me, I looked at quite a few places. There were stumbling blocks along the way as agents came to their own conclusions about my ability to run a shop. I could always tell what they were thinking as soon as they laid eyes on me. Some thought I wouldn't be able to afford the space. Others very quickly made up their mind not to lease to me. None of them wanted to take the time to understand the nature of the business or the fact that I had a track record of maintaining clients and managing my own resources. Sometimes I'd ring up an estate agent only to be told the space was taken. Later on, I'd see the 'To Let' sign still staked into the ground. I swallowed a lot of pride in those days. As upset as I was, I couldn't show it. I had to keep it moving, especially if I wanted to find the right place. I knew I would.

It's funny looking back at it now, the place I eventually chose was such a dump when I first found it. It sold household goods from around the world, but the floors and shop front had a bad paint job. I immediately had a vision of what I wanted the space to look like. I would paint the whole shop white, to bring in lots of light, and strip back the vinyl to expose the nice wooden floors underneath. I planned to also bring in details native to my Ghanaian culture, such as our wooden bowls or the Afro combs framed behind glass. When considering the property, I went to see my pastor at the time, who prophesied a shop on a strategic corner. I'd not said a word to him about the space, and so his words affirmed the acquisition for me. Then, some five years later, the landlord revealed that a hundred years ago or so the building used to be a chapel, and I knew, deep down, that it was all meant to be.

After I signed the lease, my neighbour, an architect from Australia, was instrumental in helping me design the space. We installed plinths on the ceiling to give the place a bit more edge and put up panoramic mirrors on the walls so that I had a 360° view of my surroundings. I could see my stylists on the other side of the room, and I could see tourists and all the colourful locals passing by on Portobello Road.

HAIRSTYLES THROUGH THE AGES

Dreadlocks

Dreadlocks are not just a protective style, nor are they a trend; they are a way of life for many, a symbol of an ideology that's been linked with the divine for centuries. Although there appear to be images in ancient history depicting them among the Minoans (Cretans), dreadlocks are recorded in photographs as far back as the nineteenth century, when holy Hindu men named 'sadhus' were known to lock their hair, which they called 'jatta'. According to the photographers Francesco Mastalia and Alfonse Pagano, authors of *Dreads*, the British were known to bring East Indian migrants to Jamaica as field labourers to tend profitable crops like coffee, cocoa and sugar. It's possible the natives were exposed to dreads as early as the end of the nineteenth century, with the matted locs of the sadhus a visible sign of the contract they had with the god Shiva (the destroyer and the re-creator of the universe). Their locs showed a commitment to the renunciation of everyday life. Contemporary sadhus still wear their hair in dreadlocks, and the length or thickness of the locs oftentimes reveal how long a man or a woman has been practising. Sadhus wear their hair long or tie their locs up into majestic buns or turbans 'as if to keep the true power of the hair under wraps'.[3] Mastalia and Pagano also state that other groups across India use dreadlocks to show that 'the wearer is touched by the spirit – a mystic or madman, a shaman or saint. Certain sects of Sikhism, for example, have rules directly related to kesh. Long hair indicates harmonious living, while short or shorn hair is seen as an act of disobedience, a questioning of God's will.'[4]

Mammy Wata (Water) is another popular figure, this time in Nigerian culture, whose hair is often described as long and twisted. She is known as a water spirit whose beauty is unrivalled, with her dreadlocks (or 'dada', as the style is known to the Igbo people) signifying abundance, fertility and sexuality. The significance of matted hair in Nigeria seems to differ, depending on the context. Women typically have their hair done in neat and intricate styles, often braided and away from the face. Any woman or man who leaves their hair unkempt and matted would be seen as mentally unwell or grieving, or else someone who can conjure spirits, or who has been born with divine status, such as the 'dada' children who come out of the womb with matted hair. The connection between dreadlocks and spirituality resonates across many cultures, from the Kikuyu soldiers during the Mau Mau Revolt against the British in the 50s to the Maasai warriors of Kenya who often dyed their locks red.

In more popular culture, dreadlocks are often associated with the Rastafarian religion which gained influence through political activist Marcus Garvey in the 1930s. Garvey was Jamaican-born and lived in New York City, where he founded the Universal Negro Improvement Association before deportation from the States for his radical views. He preached liberation and freedom for the Black man and stressed the importance of Africa as the Black man's origins. In Jamaica, he prophesied the rise of Ras Tafari, otherwise known as Emperor Haile Selassie I of Ethiopia, otherwise known as the 'King of Kings, Lord of Lords, Conquering Lion of the Tribe of Judah',[5] who took on mythic status for many Rastafarians who believed the Bible had foreseen his rise. Ethiopia suddenly became a promised land ruled by a chosen king. During Selassie's reign, the Lion of Judah decorated the Ethiopian flag, and the image of the animal's mane remains a longstanding symbol of the radical hairstyle. When the country was invaded by the Italians in 1935, and Selassie exiled, warriors refused to cut their locs until Selassie took back control of the throne. Rastafarians also took guidance from the scriptures when it came to the growing and maintaining of their hair. The book of Numbers 6: 5, for example, describes the tenets of the Nazarites, stating that, 'All the days of his vow of separation no razor shall come upon his head; until the time is completed for which he separates himself to the Lord, he shall be holy; he shall let the locks of hair of his head grow long.'

Although the Rastafarian theology preaches love, peace and brotherhood, it arose as a backlash against imperialist power and control in the Caribbean. It strove to put the Black man back at the centre of his destiny, as well as to preach a sense of self-love. British colonialists attempted to stifle the movement, which they saw as encroaching on their power and control through its political messages of sovereignty taken from Garvey's Black Power Movement. There are many ideas about where the origins of the word 'dreadlock' comes from. According to Ayana Byrd and Lori Tharps, the term comes from the word 'dreadful', which was used to describe the state of the matted locks seen on slaves after months of being held on ships. The term dreadlock is also speculated to have been used as a derogatory word by the British to describe a hairstyle they saw as wild, scary and untameable, but like any word used to denigrate a people, it was reclaimed and used as a source of pride. It's no surprise then that Rastafarians began to see themselves as crusaders in a foreign land. Some people today tend to spell dreadlock without the 'a' to avoid its past meaning.

The 40s and 50s saw the biggest boom in the spreading of Rastafarianism, with men beginning to preach the divinity of Ras Tafari, gathering believers and creating communities on compounds, which were later raided by the authorities. Supporters locked their hair after seeing images of Ethiopian warriors who wore dreadlocks during the Italian invasion, and pictures of Selassie as a child with matted hair. According to the Jamaican anthropologist Michael Garfield Smith, men who adhered to the scriptures religiously were called Locksmen. They kept their hair and beards in the traditional dreadlock style, never cutting or altering its growth. They viewed their actions as a sacrifice and testament to their purity as they were often ridiculed and rejected from society, or punished for their beliefs. The unimpeded growth of their hair was seen as being in harmony with nature, its abundance often compared to a flowering tree. The Beardsmen, however, were seen as dead trees without leaves because, although they grew their hair, they occasionally trimmed it and did not lock it. There were, of course, Rastafarians who did not subscribe to the hairstyle due to the prevailing negative attitudes and the inability to find or keep work.

The 70s brought on yet another boom in the hairstyle, with Bob Marley (and other reggae artists) popularizing the look through his own relationship with Rastafarianism and the spreading of his beliefs through music. The power and presence of Marley inspired many young people across cultures, races and ethnicities to adopt the iconic style.

LOCS

More people are choosing to wear locs, a healthy and gorgeous choice for our hair. Locs make a powerful statement about our race and our natural beauty. Women and men who wear them feel their hair is sacred, but the style is also worn these days as a fashion or beauty statement, from faux locs (using extensions to create the look) to funky dreads (shaving the sides of the head and palm rolling the hair at the top). The style gets its name from the locking process that occurs when hair is not combed, brushed or manipulated, causing strands to intertwine permanently. Locticians (hair stylists who specialize in creating and maintaining locs) have created several techniques to achieve a polished and fabulous look.

Hand coil or palm roll

Average styling time: Approximately 4 hours, depending on hair length

Style duration: Permanent

The hand coil method is best used on smaller-sized locs as opposed to medium or larger locs, which are more suited to the palm roll. Both methods require dividing the hair into small sections and using a water-soluble gel to either twirl each section between your index finger and thumb (hand coil) or roll each section between the base of both palms (palm roll). Continue to twirl or roll the hair until the strand ends. The most difficult part of the process is the beginning. Hair cannot be washed vigorously until it begins to lock together, which can take six to eight weeks, depending on the texture of your hair. The thicker your hair is, the faster it will lock, so this is something to take into consideration. Until you are able to shampoo thoroughly, cleanse your scalp with cotton swabs dipped in rose water and spray your scalp with a mixture of water and oils.

FAUX LOCS

Faux locs (with crochet braids)

Average styling time: 4 hours

Style duration: 4 to 6 weeks

Faux locs (twisted)

Average styling time: 4 hours

Style duration: 4 to 6 weeks

Although the maintenance of traditional dreadlocks can be a spiritual and nourishing experience, they require a certain level of time and commitment, not to mention the desire to feel more connected to a higher power. If you fancy the look of dreadlocks but are afraid to commit to the real thing, faux locs are a great option and serve as another protective style that entails using extensions to cover up your natural hair. It's a great style for women who are transitioning from relaxed to natural hair, and it's a way to get dreadlocks without having to make a permanent decision.

Faux locs are on trend, but the hairstyle can cause tension at the root of the hair due to the amount of extensions needed. This can lead to hair breakage if the extensions are too heavy, and the weight of the additional hair can cause neck pain. These are all things to consider before braving the look. There are two ways to achieve the style, either by box braiding or cornrowing. Before applying the extensions, make sure your hair is properly washed, conditioned and moisturized, indulging in a hair mask or deep treatment beforehand.

Method one: crochet braiding

Tools you will need

- Latch-hook crochet needle
- Human hair, synthetic hair or Marley braids
- A tail comb or a metal dreading comb with wooden handles
- Hair oil for scalp and edges

Step by step

1. Section and braid the hair depending on how small or large you want the locs to be. The way you section the hair also depends on how you want to wear the final style, whether that be with a side parting to the left or right or a middle parting, etc.
2. Take your crochet needle (making sure the hook at the end is closed) and insert it into the base of one of the braids.
3. Take one of the loc extensions by the loop at the base. Open the hook of the crochet needle and thread the loop of the extension inside the hook before closing.

4. Weave the base of the loc (now in the crochet needle) through the base of the braid. Afterwards, take the needle out and hold the loc of hair by the loop in one hand.
5. Hold the braid and the body of the loc in the other hand, pulling both through the loop of the extension. Make sure to pull tightly to secure.
6. Gently unravel the loc and start wrapping the braid around the loc in the direction that the extension naturally twists. Make sure to wrap the braid tightly around the loc, especially at the root, to prevent the braid from showing.
7. Twist the braid around the extension until the braid is fully immersed.
8. Begin again with the other braided sections of hair, until finished with the entire head.

Method two: cornrowing

A faster way to create the above look is to cornrow your natural hair first and then crochet the loc extensions into the rows. Installation can take anywhere between three to six hours, depending on whether you're doing it at home, with a professional, the amount of natural hair you're working with, etc.

Faux locs maintenance

Maintaining faux locs is incredibly easy and involves gently washing the hair once a week and allowing the hair to air-dry. Depending on the amount of hair added, it might be faster to use a blow-dryer or a hooded dryer at home or in the salon. Throughout the maintenance of the style, it is crucial to keep the scalp moisturized with oils. It's a good idea to wrap your locs at night to keep them looking neat and to prevent unravelling. Hair should be retwisted every four to six weeks.

ALTERNATIVES TO FAUX LOCS

If you're looking for something a little less alternative than faux locs, two strand twists and box braids are both excellent options to achieve. Hair extensions can be used to create the simple two or three strand twists, which can be worn long like dreads and can vary in width, from small to chunky, depending on your desired look.

Two strand twists

Average styling time: 2 hours for natural hair; 4–6 hours with extensions

Style duration: 2 weeks for natural hair; 4–6 weeks with extensions

Two strand twists are also known as kinky twists, Senegalese twists or twist braids. It's a method of styling hair that can incorporate hair extensions into existing natural hair for a longer look. The style involves taking two strands of hair and winding or twisting them tightly around each other until the very end. The style can be a bit more playful by unravelling the twist from the ends after a period of time, using a moisturizer on your fingers as you work through each twist, to define the wave and add more texture. You can have any style, regardless of length and colour. However, this style takes time and patience to achieve.

TIPS & TRICKS

How to do two strand twists

Tools you will need

- Tail comb
- Synthetic or natural extensions
- Pomade for edges
- Jug of hot water

Step by step

1. Part a small square section of hair.
2. Divide the squared section into two equal strands.
3. Take a small section of hair from the pack of extensions.
4. Fold your extensions in half and place the centre of the extension in between the two strands.
5. Combine one side of the folded extension with one strand of natural hair and do the same using the other side of the folded extension. You will now have two strands, each with a bit of natural hair and the extension.

6. Twist the right strand about an inch and do the same with the left strand. Make sure to twist both strands towards the right.

7. Continue twisting the strands, making sure they are firm. Then fold the right strand over the left until you have worked your way down.

8. Continue twisting until your natural hair disappears and you've reached the end of the extension.

9. Dip hair into hot water (be careful) to seal the ends together and to keep the braids looking uniform.

Box braids

Average styling time: 4 hours

Style duration: 6 to 8 weeks

Braids have always been popular with women with Type 4C hair because they afford a certain level of freedom. Women can work out, sweat or even swim, without worrying about the repercussions of shrinkage and maintenance. Braids come in all shapes and sizes and there are many styles and techniques to employ, such as two strand twists (Senegalese), micro-braids (very small single braids) and cornrows (braids attached to the scalp). Braids can be achieved with human or synthetic hair, although the former is the most desirable as it tends to look more natural and is gentler on the scalp. Braids should be washed weekly as dirt and product build-up accumulate quickly in the hair. The hair at the scalp should also be washed and involves lightly massaging the scalp with a moisturizing shampoo. It's best to use gentle movements to avoid friction and frizziness at the roots. Always remember that when you're wearing braids (or locs or any other protective hairstyle) it's important to massage the scalp with a light oil. A good massage with the fingers in a circular motion increases blood circulation and stimulates the natural flow of oil from your scalp to the rest of your hair.

Braids can be refreshed every four weeks, especially at the front, and then rebraided to protect the hairline. Braids can be worn anywhere between six and eight weeks, depending on your needs, but should be restyled to incorporate new growth and to prevent your natural hair from tangling into the extensions. Hair that's fine and straight may loosen faster than curlier, kinkier textures. Wearing braids for long periods of time can cause hair loss and damage, so it's advisable to wear your hair naturally, if you can, from time to time.

The biggest factor to note when wearing braids is the possibility of traction alopecia. Braids should never be painful when being applied, and hair should never be tugged or pulled tightly. If you ever notice bumps or small white pimples on the scalp or experience itchiness, redness or soreness, and a generally very tender scalp, braids should be removed immediately as these are all symptoms of traction alopecia. Although it is possible to do box braids on your own, most women prefer having them done by an expert braider for ease and efficiency.

TIPS & TRICKS

How to do box braids

Tools you will need

- Tail comb
- Human hair or synthetic hair
- Pomade for edges
- Jug of hot water

Step by step

1. Part a small square section of hair.
2. Take a similar section of hair from the pack of extensions.
3. Fold your extensions in half and place the centre of the extension in between the section of hair.
4. Begin braiding all three strands until the natural hair disappears.
5. Gather a bit of hair from the two other strands to create a third strand.
6. Braid until the end.
7. Dip hair into hot water (be careful) to seal the ends together and to keep the braids looking uniform.

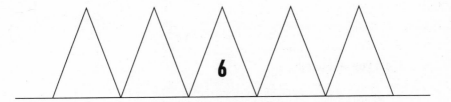

6

THE GOLDEN YEARS

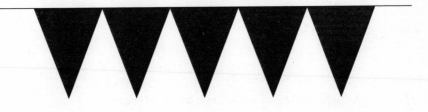

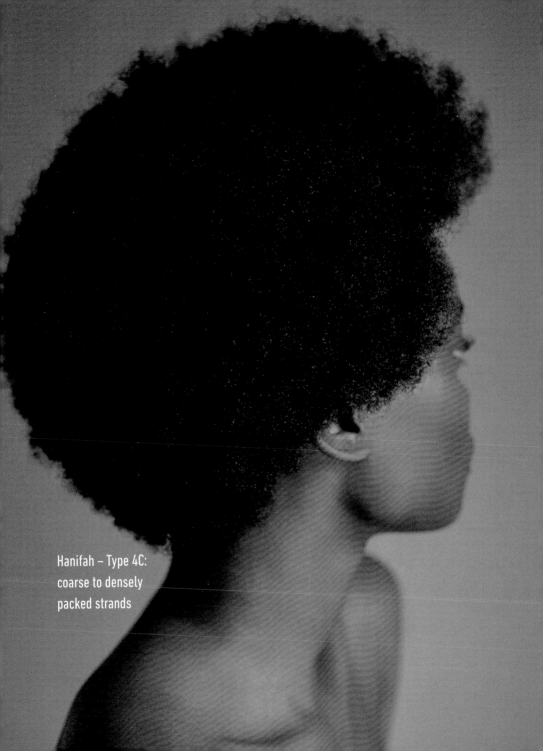

Hanifah – Type 4C:
coarse to densely
packed strands

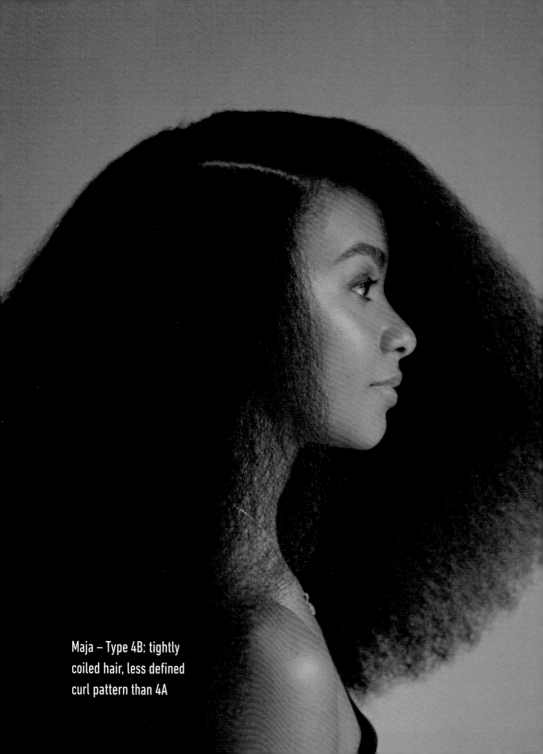

Maja – Type 4B: tightly coiled hair, less defined curl pattern than 4A

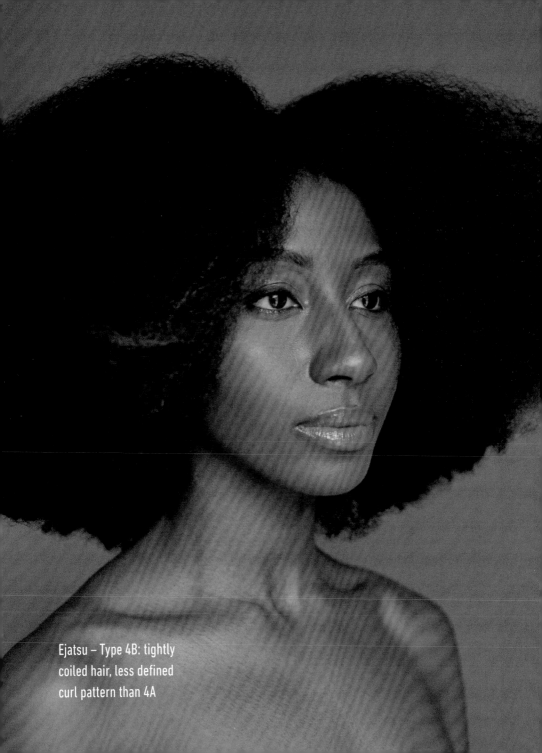

Ejatsu – Type 4B: tightly
coiled hair, less defined
curl pattern than 4A

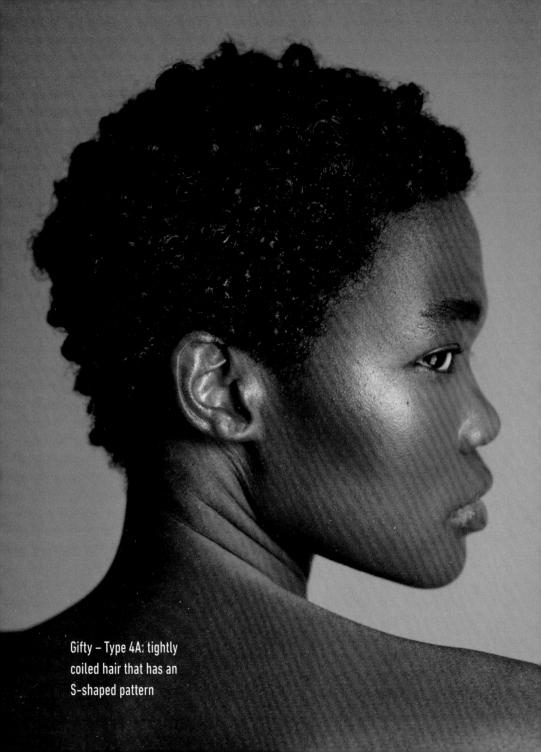

Gifty – Type 4A: tightly coiled hair that has an S-shaped pattern

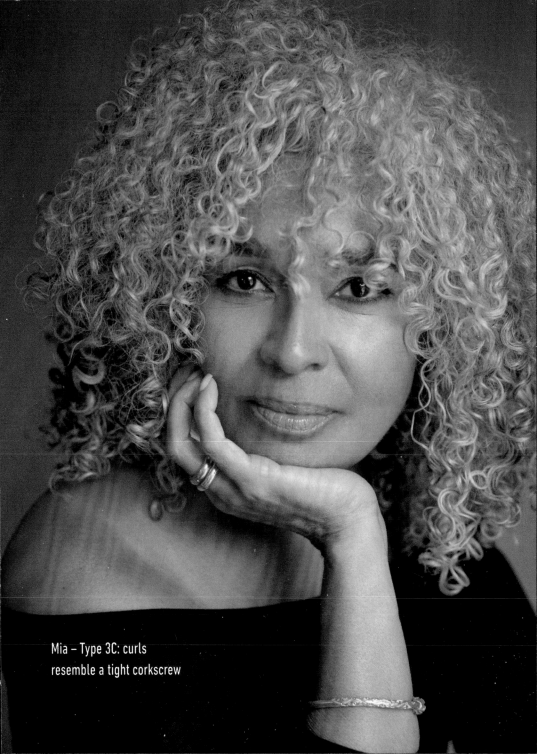

Mia – Type 3C: curls
resemble a tight corkscrew

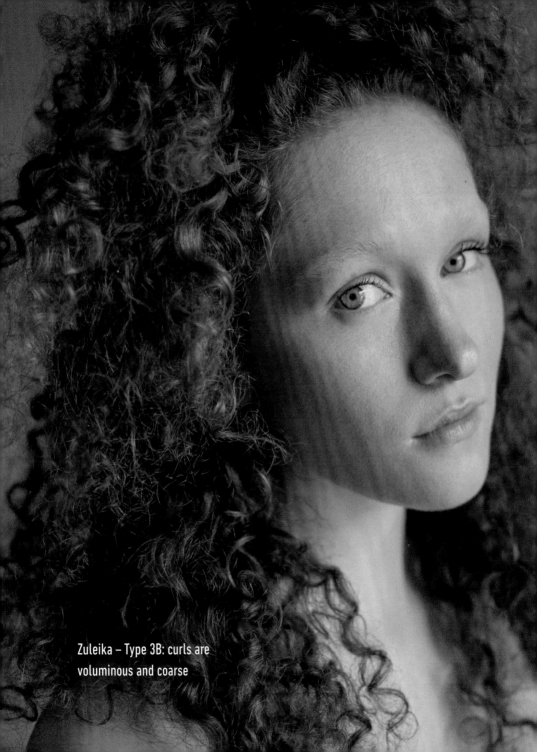

Zuleika – Type 3B: curls are
voluminous and coarse

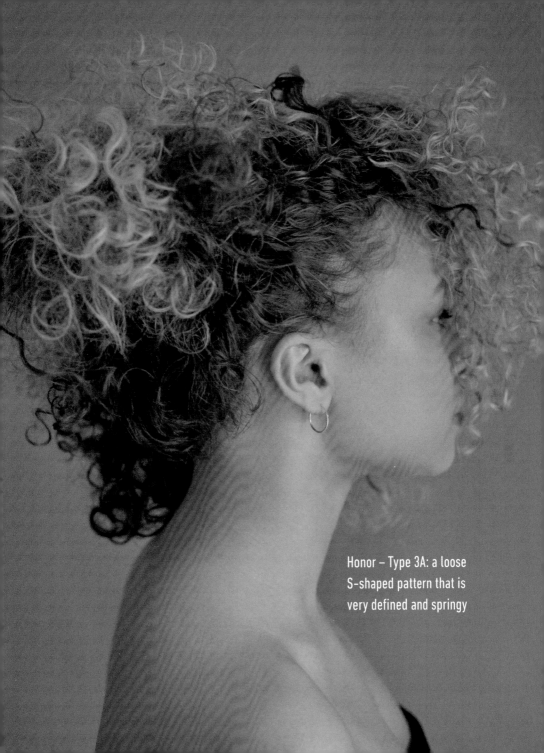

Honor – Type 3A: a loose
S-shaped pattern that is
very defined and springy

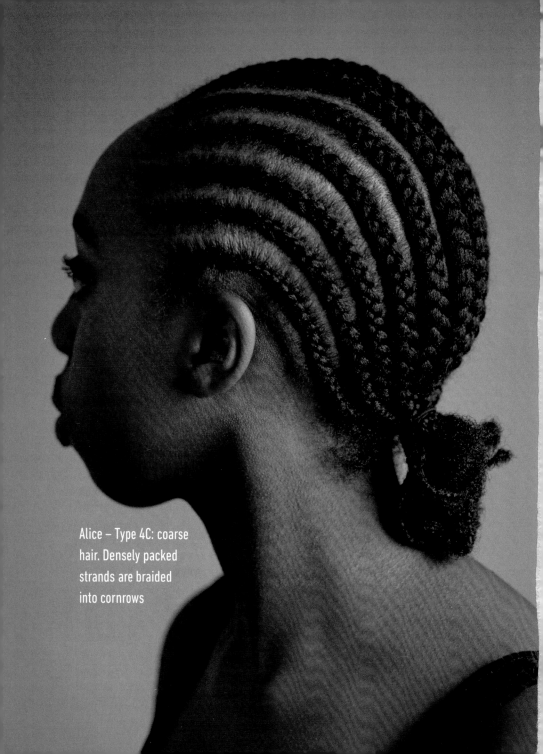

Alice – Type 4C: coarse hair. Densely packed strands are braided into cornrows

A BRIEF HISTORY OF BLACK FEMALE ENTREPRENEURSHIP

Madam C. J. Walker is probably the most well-known figure of early Black female entrepreneurship. She represented a brand of feminism that not only uplifted Black women but shattered stereotypes about the role of gender and race in society. In her early years, her story is one of strife and endurance. Walker was born Sarah Breedlove in Louisiana in 1867, at the end of the American Civil War, to emancipated slaves Owen and Minerva Breedlove. They raised six children in a small shack while continuing to pick cotton on a plantation. When Sarah was seven years old she lost her parents, and at the age of fourteen she married her first husband. Then by the age of twenty, she became a widow, left to raise a young child.

Breedlove and her daughter, Leila, moved to St Louis where they began to attend church. Many of the women in the congregation were middle-class Black women who enjoyed keeping their hair straight and 'neat' as a reflection of their class background. Sarah took up work as a laundress and, around this time, began to suffer hair loss. She strove to create a product that would assist in its regrowth. Haircare products at the time were mostly created and sold by white men capitalizing on the damaging stereotypes and popular misconceptions of Afro hair. Many of the products were aimed at straightening the hair and conforming to European standards of beauty. The formulas were toxic and mostly made for financial benefit rather than the health of the hair. Black women were also creating their own recipes at home, but it was Madam C. J. Walker (as she later named herself) who became known for launching her products on a larger scale.

Walker spent two years working for Annie Turnbo Malone, another successful Black female entrepreneur, responsible for creating the Poro Company, a haircare brand that hired agents to sell her products door to door, much like the Avon company (or the California Perfume Company, as it was called then). Malone's products would go on to sell all over the United States and across the world, from the Caribbean to Latin America. Her business strategy, which included training and certifying Black female entrepreneurs in the use of her products, would become central to Walker's own business plan. Malone also offered training courses and encouraged women to open their own Poro salons.

During the two years Walker spent as a saleswoman for the Poro Company, she honed her craft and started the long process of making and testing her own products. Walker claimed that the inspiration for the ingredients in her successful Hair Grower came from a dream, although it's been revealed that the ingredients of the Poro Company Hair Grower (petrolatum, beeswax and sulphur) were more than likely the source for her products.

Walker was a politically conscious and charismatic business-woman who wanted to distance herself from the middle-class women of her church, obsessed with straighter looks. She labelled herself a 'hair culturalist', someone interested in the growth of the hair rather than its taming. In 1906, Walker moved to Denver and launched her own brand, travelling and selling her products all over the United States. Her sales pitch compared the tending of a garden with its grass and soil to the maintenance of the hair and scalp. She later employed women on low incomes as sales agents, training them to act as missionaries who went door to door to convert men and women to using her Black-owned products. Her marketing strategy was more successful than that of her white counterparts as she used herself and the health of her hair as a model for what her products could do, and it was refreshing for Black men and women to see another dark-skinned face at the heart of the brand.

THE WALKER BRAND

Although Walker stressed the health of Afro hair, drawing on her own issues with hair loss, she still catered to the demands of what men and women wanted at the time: straight and 'manageable' hair. Walker is often falsely known for creating the hot comb to straighten Afro hair. Instead, she's one of the many people who introduced the tool to Black audiences. The Hair Grower was her bestselling product, but she also created shampoos and pomades.

Her target market for her products were Southern migrants, but as a savvy businesswoman she aimed to attract the attention of prominent Black leaders and institutions across the church, politics and women's clubs, and 'Walker's extensive outreach started to pay dividends. In 1908, two years after branching out on her own, she was earning close to $7,000 annually. The next year, she banked close to $9,000, the equivalent of over $200,000 when compared to incomes in 2015.'[1]

THE STORY OF MY MANKETTI OIL PRODUCTS

There are lots of products out there for Afro-Caribbean hair that are overwhelmingly cosmetic, synthetic or have tacky packaging. It's also a struggle to find retailers with the knowledge to effectively advise and recommend. I wanted to build a brand that embodied my beliefs and introduce a new kind of product to the market that would stand the test of time. My own journey was six years in the making. It began with the idea of importing and selling shea butter, way before the product showed up in all our household products, from oils to loo roll. I planned to package the butter in the calabash, a gourd found in West Africa, but when I tried bringing them through customs, I was told they were restricted items because of their composition! They were not as durable as I thought and wouldn't stand the test of extreme heat or cold. By the time I found a more modern solution to the packaging, shea butter had lost its edge.

The discovery of my active ingredient didn't come to me in a dream, nor did it come from anything I had ever known before. Instead, it came in 2010, when I was asked to work at a wedding in the Serengeti in East Africa. After a nine-hour trip chock-full of transfers, and styling the next day, I was due a hard-earned massage. Hairdressing isn't all chatting and laughter and glamour. Sometimes it's a bad back and shoulders and very tired legs. The therapist massaged my skin and hair with a mysterious oil that melted into my skin and left my hair looking and feeling great. She told me it was Manketti Oil which came from the mongongo nut indigenous to southern regions of Africa, such as Namibia and Botswana, and surrounding areas. From that moment on, I knew I needed to get my hands on that oil, which I later learned contained high levels of polyunsaturated fat, a good building block for nourishment. Not only was the oil moisturizing, it was incredibly lightweight. I researched the people of Namibia and their history and grew more and more fascinated by the day. I knew from the get-go that creating my own brand would go deeper than financial gain, and the idea that I could help communities by buying what belonged to them felt absolutely right.

Manketti Oil became a secret I had to keep to myself for years. I had discovered a miracle and needed to get everything locked down, from the licensing to the sourcing. It then took some time to find the right chemist. I needed to work with someone I connected with, someone who knew or wanted to know more about Afro hair. Six chemists later, I finally found the one, and we developed a lovely working relationship. Luckily for me, having the salon meant that I could test the products as he experimented, experiencing the results on different hair types. Clients could return after using a sample and report on the product's longevity in terms of moisture.

The years I had spent consulting for big brands pushed me to further refine my own brand. It took many years of trial and error, and timing, to get the story of the packaging and products right. There's a whole person in a brand, and that requires a strong sense of self. I found myself packaging my heritage and livelihood in one bottle, bringing the best of both my worlds, from London to Accra. The shapes found on my products' boxes and bottles are inspired by the patterns found on Ghanaian Kente cloth. My grandparents used to adorn themselves in the material during family gatherings, which always made them look very regal. I was also inspired by the Kuba cloth of Sierra Leone, a mud cloth, handwoven in uneven cubes and graphic shapes, which is the inspiration behind the initials on the packaging. Finally, the gold lettering represents the richness of African soil and harks back to the days when Ghana was known as the Gold Coast.

THE BRITISH HAIRDRESSING AWARDS

My name on the map

A few years after establishing the Hair Lounge on Portobello Road, I needed to attract more customers. My clientele already consisted of women who had come to see me at home or at the business centre in Kilburn, and there were those who I flew to visit on big occasions like weddings, which I seemed to be doing once or twice a month across Europe, Africa and the Caribbean. All of this was well and good, but I was itching to start a new project to get my name on the map. I approached the editor of *Black Hair* magazine about writing a column on natural hair. There wasn't much written about natural hair or styles here in the UK; you only heard about the phenomenon in America, where there seemed to be a big movement happening. In the early 2000s, nine out of ten women who rang the salon were calling to get a relaxer or a weave. Yet here I was, going in the opposite direction, trying to get women to adopt more natural hairstyles. So, when I had the opportunity to create a how-to column every six weeks, the project felt like the boost I needed to continue spreading the word about the beauty of our natural hair.

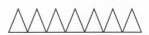

In the early 2000s, nine out of ten women who rang the salon were calling to get a relaxer or a weave. Yet here I was, going in the opposite direction, trying to get women to adopt more natural hairstyles.

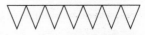

We called the column 'Natural Fix'. It was a hair clinic of sorts – a client would come to the salon looking for an update, rather than just to be pampered. I would then have a chat during the consultation stage and find out more about them: what kind of job they did, what sort of places they liked to go, whether they were a student or a working professional, whether they worked in a creative environment or someplace more corporate. Some people are quirky, and you can see it in their dress sense, and you know straight away that they'll want to do something more daring. Others are more conservative and reserved, so their look needs to be clean and structured. First impressions matter a lot, as well as communication. Many women know what they want from the get-go. Maybe they've seen a picture in a magazine or a celebrity on the red carpet sporting a new do. We profiled clients by name, age and occupation, stated their 'Problem' and came up with a 'Solution'. I took the reader through the 'Process' of achieving the new look in six easy steps. We provided photos of each phase of styling, as well as a 'before' and 'after' picture, so readers could see the transformation. Oftentimes, it felt like looking at a completely different woman, and it inspired a lot of new clients who read the magazine and thought, 'If she can do that to her hair, what can she do for me?'

Writing the columns for 'Natural Fix' led to me being more and more creative. I learned to come up with quick solutions for the men and women who came to me wanting to have their hair styled in a natural way. The key to convincing women to wear more natural styles began with me. I had to be confident enough to pull off a certain look as soon as they sat in my chair. If I could show them a style that suited the shape of their face, the sort of products that worked best for their hair type, and talk them through how to look after their hair properly, then they would feel more encouraged to wear a more natural look instead of putting their hair in braids or wearing a wig. One thing I had going for me in terms of inspiration was the location of my shop on Portobello Road. It's probably the most eclectic and happening place in London, and all sorts of stylish people pass by. I used to look at a lot of magazines for research, tweaking what I found with my own little twist. My everyday clients were my biggest influence, people who told me about where they were going and where they had been. Their stories motivated and pushed me to do something different every time.

Looking back, the coming together of my interactions with clients and my 'Natural Fix' columns gave me the conviction and confidence to start entering hair competitions. In 2013, I assembled my first 'Texture' collection for the Afro Hair category of the British Hairdressing Awards, otherwise known as the 'Oscars of hairdressing'. I studiously analysed past entries in the category and thought about ways I could bring something new to the table. My first collection was a response to past entries I'd seen over the years, which all rehashed the same old androgynous or avant-garde images. On top of this, the textures failed to reflect our natural curl patterns. I wanted to set the bar high, to create collections that were elegant using traditional hairstyles. I wanted to use Black models who exuded serenity instead of the sexualized imagery that I was seeing a lot of. The competitions forced me out of my comfort zone, and in doing so I had to make a statement: 'This is me. This is what I stand for. This is what I think Afro hair looks like.'

I spent the next five years developing a signature look, but this took time and loads of money. I needed to pay models and photographers, make-up artists and assistants, and buy time in the studio. Some years I couldn't afford it, and other years I saved months in advance. I knew that even if I didn't win a competition, the platform was still a great place to showcase my work. I could create these beautiful images and later publish them in magazines around the world. It was a great way for people to know my name and to publicize my work, not only to my peers but to potential clients later.

If you're an aspiring hairdresser looking to eventually enter the competitions, it's essential to plan the collections at least a year ahead of time. January is spent finalizing your concept and by April you're sourcing models and putting together budgets. By May you're submitting your first collection and awaiting the results. If you've made it to the next round, you're submitting a second collection in September, with winners announced at the end of November. Having a definitive concept for the shoot is the most important part of the process. If you don't know exactly what you're doing or what you're trying to say, then what's the point? It's very important to know what it is you're selling. Are you selling curls or are you selling natural hair? What's the message you're trying to communicate?

My second collection entered the finals and won. My photographer and I created silhouettes that played with light and shade, and this gave the hair of my models a luminous and ethereal quality. My second collection the following year (2014) also won. The concept took inspiration from the glamorous hairstyles of the 70s but pushed the familiar boundaries much further. It was this collection that brought me a great friend and collaborator, John Rawson, an amazing photographer whose vision for the collection aligned directly with my own, so much so that on the first day we met, we both discovered that we'd saved the same inspirational image on the home screens of our phones. The second collection brought many new opportunities, including working with Pepsi and Janelle Monáe on the 2014 Brazilian World Cup campaign. I also began consulting for big brands during this time, such as the L'Oréal brand Mizani. They were creating a new range called True Textures, for natural hair, and asked me to be the brand ambassador responsible for all the styling and the shoots. We were able to secure Shingai Shoniwa from the band Noisettes to be the new face of the products. True Textures became one of L'Oréal's highest-selling products at the time and I believe they were the first company to really go deep and produce a range for Black Afro hair.

I would say that my most memorable invitation after winning my second collection came from the Aveda Congress, a biannual celebration of hair featuring all the Aveda network worldwide. The committee asked me to put on a thirty-minute show of my work in front of an audience in Minneapolis, Minnesota. When I showed up, I took one look at the size of the auditorium and thought, 'I can't do this. I'm too shy!' Imposter syndrome is a real thing; even with all my success I felt like I didn't deserve to be there. But when it came to showtime, I sought to connect the audience with my work and myself. I used the same playlist I used in my salon and spoke to the audience in the same way I speak to my clients. I shared stories about my life alongside hair techniques like African hair threading, which many of the stylists had never heard of or seen before. Women came up to me after the presentation in tears. Others hugged me, touched by the story of losing my mum and the journey I'd been on to get here. I had no idea at the time that sharing my life would resonate with so many, and the entire experience turned out to be more uplifting than I thought. The congress showed me a different side to hair shows.

'African Gold' (2015) was the title of my third collection. Apart from focusing on the versatility of Afro hair, I focused on the allure of skin and the aura of gold to create the ultimate standard of beauty. One of the key elements of producing the best pictures is making sure you have the right team. My photographer, John, make-up artist, Lan, and my assistants at the time were all on the same page on the day of this shoot. I led a prayer beforehand and cooked Sunday lunch for us to share. The music was right, the conversations flowing, and all the models were confirmed for the day – except one, who had yet to turn up. Four hours later, we had one hour left in the studio and no one had time to reschedule another shoot. Our pictures were also due in two weeks' time. I had already prepped this model's hair, as there's only so much you can do in a day. She was supposed to sport the shaved undercut crop look for the collection, but I wondered if I should go ahead and use one of the other models instead. When she finally turned up, we managed to finish her hair in twenty minutes and within the first five to ten minutes in front of the camera, we had the perfect shot. There were a lot of highs and lows behind that image, but in the end, we got exactly what we wanted and more. We made it to the finals with 'African Gold' but, unfortunately, we didn't take home the prize.

My last and final collection, shot in 2017, represents everything that I stand for: creativity, strength, power and femininity. I called it the 'Afrofuture' collection as it spoke of the self-assurance it takes to wear a bold look. We used styles like Bantu knots and braids to create geometric shapes and stayed away from trying to tame the hair through slicked-down styles with too much gel. I wanted to show the hair as it was in its most natural state, graphic but with a feminine softness. The collection was so good that after the announcement was made of my win, Erykah Badu emailed the next day. I saw her name pop up in my inbox and screamed, 'Is this for real?!' I then went on to work with her for the British Fashion Council Awards, where she rocked an intricate threaded style, the same sort of style I had been bullied for, as a child.

After winning three Afro hair competitions, in 2018 I became the first Black woman to be inducted into the British Hairdressing Awards Hall of Fame. The awards ceremony was a momentous occasion at one of London's landmark hotels, the Grosvenor House on Park Lane. The most striking thing for me was the impact it had on my dad, who used to work there as a dishwasher. Yet there I was on stage, fifty years later, the dishwasher's daughter celebrating my determination to make a difference and showcase the breadth and wealth of styles for Afro hair. My father broke down in tears that night when I accepted my award, but he was the one who had sowed the seeds for me to be there.

I'm now one of the seventy judges for the British Hairdressing Awards, which is such an honour and a privilege. We meet in a room full of photographs representing the work of various stylists across categories such as 'London Hairdresser of the Year' or 'Men's Hairdresser of the Year', probably the largest category in the competition. Each category has about fifteen to thirty applicants, and it's up to us to whittle it down to six. I'll usually walk into the room and be hit by the winning image, that's how automatic a feeling it is for me. The photograph must move or touch my spirit somehow. Sometimes contestants forget it's a hair competition, and there's too much going on. The hair, for me, must be the most popping thing in the image, not the earrings, not the clothing, not the make-up. I pay close attention to the health of the hair, too, and if a contestant has dyed a model's hair, I want to see that the colour has been well executed and that the hair still has integrity. I want to see that the hair looks shiny and conditioned instead of dead or fried. It's all about the details for me, and it's all about simplicity – but simple, of course, is hard to do.

CASE STUDY

Moisture mania

A client had an event coming up and wanted a new style, but her biggest problem was that her hair was very dry, lacked lustre and had no curl definition. She'd seen many positive reviews of my Manketti Oil products and wanted me to work my magic. I recommended she have regular steam treatments and suggested she go for a round, soft and curly Afro to show how versatile her hair could be.

Her hair was washed using my Manketti Oil Shampoo. This creamy shampoo instantly moisturizes and fortifies as it cleanses, leaving the hair supple and manageable. Hair was then steam treated using my oil conditioner, which replenishes lost moisture and leaves the hair feeling healthier and manageable. After a twenty-minute treatment, I rinsed off and towel-dried. One drop of Manketti Oil was applied through mid-length and ends, then blow-dried with a paddle brush to straighten out curls before cutting. Curls can often weigh down a haircut, which was the case with this client's hair. I gently took a vertical section and, with minimum tension, cut from short to long using the perimeter as a guide. I continued in this manner until the cut was complete.

I then sprayed the hair using a bottle half filled with water and a fifty-pence-piece-sized dab of Manketti Oil Conditioner and two drops of Manketti Hair Oil. I tilted the head down and held the diffuser at a 90° angle. I then lifted the roots away from the scalp and scrunched the hair until dry. (I would suggest flipping the hair back to allow it to dry naturally.) The goal of diffusing is to reduce frizz and seal in moisture and shine. Another drop of oil was applied to the client's hair to give her curls more of a pop.

TIPS & TRICKS

Manketti Oil conditioning treatments

I absolutely love making my own product cocktails and one of my favourites is a conditioning treatment I make at home which involves Manketti Oil and shea butter. I use it once a week and it makes my hair shiny and soft. It's my go-to conditioner when my hair needs a little TLC. Everybody's hair is different, but for my own I usually mix a drop of each, as this is the perfect way to nourish my hair without weighing it down.

If you're looking for a good leave-in conditioner, I suggest mixing in a spray bottle a few pumps of Manketti Oil Conditioner (depending on the length and texture of your hair) and about a quarter of a cup of water. This creates a white milky emulsion that keeps the hair nourished and refreshed. It's also a nice way to detangle curly hair, section by section, using a paddle brush before shampooing, or to keep in at night before a twist out.

Another way to use the conditioner is to make it into a mask. Add a few drops of Manketti Oil to a bit of Manketti Oil Conditioner to make a creamy paste. Slather on to your hair and cover with a plastic cap for twenty to thirty minutes, or even an hour, before washing off. The mask will deeply penetrate the hair shaft, leaving the hair incredibly soft. You can customize any of my products, whether it be the conditioner or oil, to achieve the right product for you.

AFRICAN SHEA BUTTER: PAST AND PRESENT

African shea butter is an excellent moisturizer for Afro hair. I use it often for home-made deep conditioning treatments (and for my skin as well) so I like to stock up on my trips to Ghana, both for home and the salon. Although there are lots of products claiming to be one hundred per cent shea butter, the best varieties are raw and unrefined as they contain many of the nut's nutrients, such as vitamins A and E, and fatty acids. Natural shea butter comes in different colours, from tan to white, depending on how much it's been processed. It's sensitive to heat and will melt in hot temperatures or will turn as hard as a brick in the cold, so it's best to keep it at room temperature. The fat helps to seal in moisture, making hair less frizzy and giving it lots of shine. It's a reliable option for dry and brittle Afro hair textures. Women can also use it as a heat protectant when blow-drying or pressing. Some people find the scent of the butter strong and pungent, so I recommend mixing it with an essential oil of your choice.

Shea tree preservation dates as far back as 1000 CE and has important ecological and cosmetic benefits. The trees can be found across sub-Saharan parts of Africa, with Burkina Faso, Mali and Ghana being the largest exporters of shea. Although shea has become a popular commodity, the countries that produce it have low GDPs, and many development organizations have stepped in to make sure that those who produce the stock get remunerated properly. According to the academics Marlène Elias and Judith Carney, who studied shea production in Burkina Faso, the production of the fruit has historically been controlled by women who collect the nuts, produce the butter and sell the goods in the marketplace or to traders. The way women make butter from the nut is a process passed on from one generation to the next, usually from mother to daughter. Producing the butter is a very physical process involving fermenting the fruit, extracting the nuts and then a variation of roasting, crushing, boiling and rinsing to make a paste. Much like the art and practice of African hairdressing, the production of shea butter provides a sense of camaraderie between women, especially during the kneading of the butter, where women in Burkina Faso were observed to be singing and clapping to raise spirits. Elias and Carney state that, 'Women are recognized for the quality of their butter and skilled butter makers take great pride in their reputation. In south-western Burkina Faso, butter producers offer their finest shea butter as a gift at births and weddings and as a gesture of gratitude for acts of kindness.'[2] Sadly, shea butter production is moving away from the rituals and traditions of women to the rise of big business and technological advancements.

EDUCATING THE MASSES

Madam C. J. Walker not only set up a business for the haircare of Black people across the United States, she also set up a way of helping women to embrace enterprise. She wanted Black women to move away from the low-paying domestic jobs available to them and to take up work that gave them better pay and more freedom. Walker set up conventions in which all her agents congregated annually to discuss their progress, learn more about the ever-expanding business and upcoming products. She set up beauty colleges just like businesswoman Annie Turnbo Malone. There, women could become knowledgeable beauticians. Many of these women then went on to start their own salons, all the while stocking Walker's products. The empowerment of women just like her was integral to her business acumen, and agents all across the States held chapters or clubs where they not only came together to discuss haircare and Walker products but also to heal and talk politics – a daily reality in their lives, as Black business owners and entrepreneurs were under the threat of violence due to their financial independence and freedom.

The teaching of natural haircare has been an integral part of my career for more than thirty years now, and I've had the opportunity to travel all over the world. One of my most memorable experiences took me to Tanzania, in 2014, when I worked with an ethnic haircare brand called Namaste. The focus of the class was to teach young women about haircare practices in the West and to introduce them to some of Namaste's up-and-coming products. I will never forget the woman who came to class late because she lacked money for the bus fare. She told me much later that she'd walked a distance of what felt like Manchester to London after leaving her house at 4.30 a.m. to make the 8 a.m. start! Her legs and clothes were covered in red dust by the time she joined us. The sacrifice she endured to get to the class touched me and I remember bursting into tears that evening in my hotel room, deeply affected by her determination and spirit for wanting to achieve.

I've taught Afro hair techniques in several European countries, such as Bulgaria, where I was invited to teach at the Trinity Sport & Beauty Center, in 2011. It was located across from an African embassy, where many high-profile women were looking to have their hair done in the country. The hair salon became one of the first in the country to cater to women of Afro-Caribbean descent. Prior to this, many of these women had to travel to more metropolitan cities, such as London or Paris, just to have their hair done properly.

It's important to set up these relationships with other salons, even in countries that may not have a huge Afro-Caribbean population, and I still have young adults from Eastern Europe who come to the salon for apprenticeships. One woman recently quit her job as a hotel manager just to come and study full time. Students stay between two weeks and two years to take up lessons, and stylists have come from as far away as Japan or as near as Germany. One year, I had an entire class come from California wanting to know more about Afro hair textures and maintenance. There's a trend right now in terms of European salons learning how to diversify their offering, in order to cater to all. Many women who come to the Hair Lounge from neighbouring countries do so because they don't have salons that cater to their hair type. It's important that hairdressers learn how to be good all-rounders, not just someone who specializes in braids or weaves. When studying at Splinters, we were expected to learn how to do everything so that if anyone came through the doors, we were ready, and I still expect this of my students today.

These days, whether teaching the FAME team at GHD, or at L'Oréal, one of the things I try to impress is this: play with your hair, fall in love with your hair, but don't do too much with it, because it is what it is! Once you've established a good shape by way of a salon cut, that's your style, that's your statement. My 'Curl Power' class for the L'Oréal Academy touches on how to look after Afro hair, as well as providing different style techniques to make Afro hair look and feel its best. Some students have been hairdressing for a long time and others are just starting out, so it's a great mix of people. My curriculum usually focuses on how to create curls without using heat and how to wash and condition properly. I also teach traditional African styling like threading or two strand twists, the sort of styles never taught at more traditional European parlours.

THE IMPORTANCE OF GIVING BACK

Walker succeeded in creating a million-dollar business by selling her products globally across the Americas and the Caribbean. She, along with Malone, was also incredibly generous with her funds, often donating to Black causes and universities in order to advance Black people during a time when African Americans were being lynched and denied their rights. Walker and Malone both felt their haircare products and businesses were much larger than just beauty and aesthetics. Their businesses reflected a time of betterment for their race and their gender alike, especially when leadership was a sphere deemed more suited to men. Ultimately, the Walker brand was the meeting place between beauty, politics, charity and sister-hood. Walker died in 1919, at the age of fifty-one, after reaping the benefits of her success and eventually becoming the first Black female millionaire successfully living off her own business.

My encounter with the student in Tanzania drove me to start my charity called Love Naa Densua, named after my mother who worked hard to give back to her siblings and children even when she had so little of her own. In 2018, I also launched the Charlotte Mensah Academy, which provides further education opportunities to young women in Africa. I spend a lot of time in Ghana teaching in open-air classrooms or salons across the country; I find that being mobile is more of a priority than being static. I want to reach as many people as possible and so I take my teachings to obscure places, connecting with women who can't afford an education. The Academy allows young people the opportunity to learn hair styling skills as a sustainable way of providing an income for themselves and their families. Most of my students are young adults whose parents can't afford to put them through university. The curricu-lum involves techniques from cutting to colouring, but I also teach the finer details of haircare, such as how to do a good blow-dry or how to use products properly. My biggest focus is always on how to style natural hair without resorting to chemicals. I still teach aspects of hairdressing like weaves and the proper way to apply hair extensions, but I also instill the importance of looking after our God-given textures.

If I'm coaching in a salon, I'll spend an afternoon introducing stylists to aspects of running a business. All stylists looking to set up their own salon need to know the basics, from how to communicate with clients to the sort of music that should be played, to the look and feel of the space and the environment.

TIPS & TRICKS

Weaves (hair extensions)

Average styling time: 3 hours

Style duration: 6 weeks

As a hairstylist and businesswoman, it's important to be versatile and knowledgeable about trends, even while promoting natural hair. After all, true freedom for Black women is the choice to wear their hair as they please. These days, there's no denying the popularity of weaves, with millions of pounds of hair being imported globally from countries such as China and India. Fashion designers have always loved telling a good story with their collections and, in turn, they want models to complete the look with stunning hair. Hair extensions are added by hairdressers for that extra drama and flare, making the hair look more exaggerated, as the model's normal hair is never enough. The early 90s saw the first explosion of weaves taking off amongst Black actresses, models and singers, but the adding of real or synthetic hair has probably been around for as long as the wig. It's not only models and actresses wearing weaves but also ordinary women. In 2015, the market research firm Mintel published a report on the Black haircare market in the US with this to say about the resurgence of weaves: 'Even as Black consumers showcase a variety of hairstyles and embrace their natural hair, wigs, weaves and extensions have held their ground. Black women are spending a tremendous amount on these products annually, but they remain essential among a wide range of Black haircare consumers as they fulfill the desire to switch up hair-styles while also allowing for a simple, no-fuss daily beauty and grooming routine.'[3]

TIPS & TRICKS

Brazilian weaves

They're a great way to add length and volume and can be added to all types of hair, no matter the curl type. A professional weave will look and perform like your very own hair and can be styled and cut as if it were your own. Brazilian weaves are popular because they can be bleached or dyed and even curled with a curling iron and still maintain a healthy-looking glow. Women love this brand of hair because of its texture and its ability to be both strong and durable but soft and luxurious. Options range from free flowing to a full-bodied wave, depending on the desired look and occasion. You can also go for other human or synthetic options. Less is best when it comes to the amount of hair used. Many women make the mistake of adding too much. It's important that you treat the hair as if it were your own, using good-quality hair products and sleeping with a silk pillow at night or wrapping the hair up with a silk scarf.

Weaves are expensive and best left to a hairdresser to apply. Application takes many hours and often involves complex methods including sew ins (when hair is corn-rowed to create tracks, and wefts of hair are sewn in) and interlocking (when the weft is sewn directly to the base of the scalp with a flat rolled technique). There are also clip-ins for easier application. Always try and avoid methods that require bonding glue as this destroys the hair line, causing traction alopecia or baldness. These days, more natural-looking weaves are being created for Afro hair, which doesn't have to be long and flowing but can look coily or bobbed.

Extensions can also be used to transition from relaxed to natural hair and should be worn for no longer than six to eight weeks. You might also consider visiting your stylist every two to four weeks to groom and refresh your weave. It's very important to maintain the condition of your natural hair, regardless of texture, when wearing a weave. Use conditioning treatments before, during and after your weave. I also sug-gest massaging oil into your scalp to keep it healthy, and trimming natural hair at regular intervals to keep ends healthy.

TIPS & TRICKS

Transitioning from chemical treatments

If you're currently transitioning from relaxers to natural hair, and weaves aren't for you, there are many other styling options to consider. I find more and more women are freeing themselves from chemical treatments and damage from heated tools. Many are going back to their natural hair texture and loving it, but transitioning from straight to natural hair requires patience and effort. Today there are several ways to grow your hair out of a relaxer and keep it looking healthy.

- Flat iron with thermal straighteners
- Protective styles (braids, crochet wigs, weaves, twists, cornrows)
- Roller or rod sets (this allows you to create a head full of curls to hide the bulkiness of the new growth)
- Going short (the Big Chop)

In general, I always recommend clients have a consultation with a stylist, as growing out your hair leaves you with a mixture of virgin and chemically treated hair. Most women aren't emotionally ready for the Big Chop, but managing these two different textures can be difficult to deal with. I often address the balance by setting the hair in rollers, rods or straws, depending on hair length, for a uniform look. It gives the hair an evenly defined curl, although achieving this look yourself can be time-consuming.

CASE STUDY

Relaxed and glam

Transitioning from straight to natural hair requires patience, time and effort, but sometimes this isn't available. Years ago, a woman's only choice for transitioning would've been to cut off all her relaxed hair and start with a short natural regrowth. Thankfully, this is no longer the case as there are several ways to transition while keeping the hair looking healthy and great. A model and presenter, aged twenty-four, came to the salon to have her hair done for a red-carpet event. Her hair was breaking, which happens frequently during the transition period, and she was tired of using straightening irons as she was growing her hair out of a relaxer. She wanted to try something more natural but glamorous for her big event. After our consultation, I had the perfect vintage look for her special evening.

After washing her hair with a repair shampoo that gently and effectively revived her hair, leaving it looking nourished and strong, I applied a high-performance mask throughout the roots, mid-length and ends. The mask helped to infuse protein back into her fragile and weakened hair. I left it on for fifteen minutes and then applied an oil to blow-dry her hair with a paddle-brush. I gathered her hair into a high ponytail, using wax to slick down edges and smooth away flyaways. The ponytail was twisted into a knot and pinned down. I then used a bespoke hairpiece in dark brown, which I attached to the knot, rolling it into a chignon before securing with hairpins.

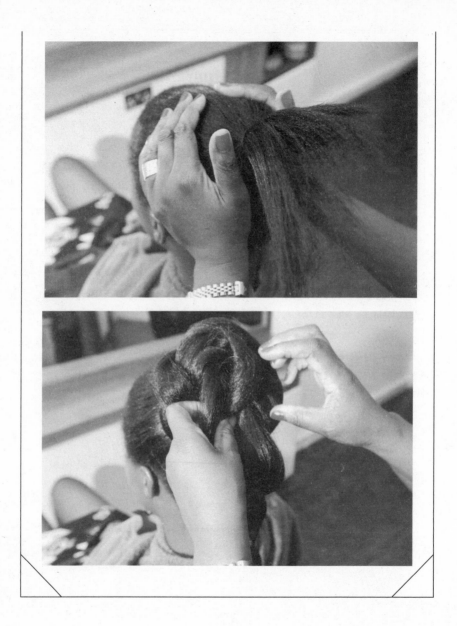

TIPS & TRICKS

What is the Big Chop?

The Big Chop involves taking your hair journey from transitioning to one hundred per cent natural in a matter of minutes! Once your hair has been relaxed it will never go back to its natural form, no matter what products you use. In order to go back to your roots, you have one option and one option only: to cut your relaxed hair and start with a TWA (Teeny Weeny Afro). Now that your hair is short, it will be easier to test out different products without having to go through the lengthy process of detangling, etc. It's best to have a professional stylist do the Big Chop for you, but if you're feeling adventurous . . .

Tools you will need

- Wide toothcomb or paddle brush
- Butterfly clips
- Hair bands
- Scissors

Step by step

1. Use a wide toothcomb or paddle brush to section off your freshly washed hair into four large sections.
2. Apply butterfly clips to keep each section separated.

3. Put each section into a mini ponytail with a band so the line of demarcation is exposed above the hair band. The demarcation line is the weakest point on each strand, making it extremely vulnerable to breakage.

4. Once your entire head has been sectioned off into bands, cut off your relaxed hair.

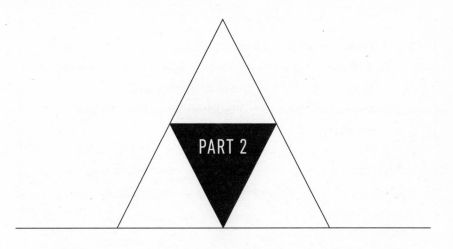

PART 2

GOOD HAIR: HOW TO CARE FOR YOUR HAIR

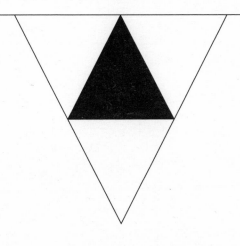

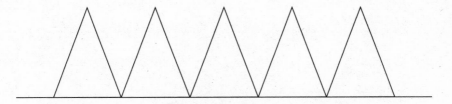

GLOSSARY

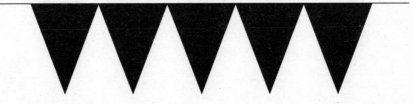

Afro – A hairstyle consisting of very tight curls which grow outwardly.

Alopecia – Hair loss or baldness on the scalp or any place on the body where hair grows.

Alopecia areata – Round, bald patches on the scalp or anywhere on the body.

Alopecia totalis – Baldness affecting the entirety of the scalp.

Alopecia universalis – Hair loss affecting the entirety of the scalp and body.

Anagen – The first and most active phase of the human hair growth cycle, where the hair grows for 1,000 days or more.

Bantu knots – Individual braids or twisted hair spun around itself to form a tight knot or coil. Originated from South African Zulus.

Beehive – Big, poofy hair bun, popular in the 60s.

Big Chop – Taking your hair journey from transitioning to one hundred per cent natural in one go by cutting off all relaxed hair.

Bonded glue extensions – A weave technique applied to the whole or partial head. They are attached directly to the root of the client's hair and therefore sit flatter on the head than a sewn weave.

Box braids – Thick braids that are added to natural hair using synthetic or human hair extensions.

Braids – Loose hair made up of three interlaced strands that move freely. This is usually done with human or synthetic hair. They can be any width or length.

Catagen – The second or transitional stage of the human hair growth cycle, which involves the shrinkage of hair follicles and hair becoming loosely attached.

Clarifying and cleansing shampoo – A type of shampoo that lifts residues and environmental pollutants from the hair.

Colour conditioner – Maintains the vibrancy of your hair colour after the use of hair dye and should be used after every wash.

Conditioner – A liquid product used after a shampoo to moisturize the hair, making it soft and manageable when combing or brushing.

Conditioning shampoo – Used to treat dry, brittle and damaged hair as well as chemically treated and colour-processed hair.

Cornrows (or canerows) – A three-strand braiding technique attached to the scalp in rows.

Cortex – The middle layer of the hair shaft, found between the medulla and the cuticle.

Co-washing – Using conditioner to wash the hair instead of shampoo.

Crochet braids – A method of adding synthetic or human hair extensions to natural, cornrowed hair using a latch-hook crochet needle.

Curly perm (or Jheri curl) – A hairstyle achieved using a chemical treatment called ammonium thioglycolate. The process involves chemically straightening the hair before the application of perm rods, for a looser curl.

Cuticle – The outermost layer of the hair, made of overlapping protective sheaths.

Dandruff – A dry and itchy scalp condition that results in flaking skin.

Deep penetrating conditioners – Conditioners that should be used once a month or every two weeks, depending on the condition of the hair, especially after braids and extensions are removed.

Dermis – The middle layer of the skin.

Diffuser – Bowl-shaped attachments that disperse the flow of air from your blow-dryer.

Dreadlocks – Hair that is rolled or twisted into locs that allow the hair to grow without too much manipulation or grooming.

Dye – Chemical treatments used to change your natural hair colour or to cover up grey hair.

Edges – The shortest hair on the head that usually grows from the front of the hairline.

Emollient – A cream or liquid that soothes and softens the skin.

End papers – Square-cut fibre papers used to gather the ends of the hair when using rods, rollers or straws.

Epidermis – The uppermost layer of the skin.

Extensions – Hair that is added to natural hair to add volume or length. Can be 'natural' or synthetic (for example, Kanekalon, which is often used for braids); come in all colours, textures and lengths.

Flat iron – A tool usually made of ceramic or metal plates that, when heated, straightens the hair, temporarily changing its structure.

Hair bulb – The base of the hair follicle, where the hair is still alive.

Hair follicle – Small holes all over the surface of human skin that grow hair.

Hair porosity – The hair's ability to absorb and keep moisture. Fine hair tends to be more porous, whereas coarse hair is not.

Hair shaft – The part of the hair seen on the surface of the skin and scalp, divided into three sections: the medulla, cortex and cuticle.

Hair supplements – support healthy growth from within. They commonly contain antioxidants such as vitamins A, C and E.

Hot comb – A combing tool made of metal, often heated on a stove (or electrically wired), to temporarily straighten Afro hair.

Humectant – A substance that maintains or seals in moisture.

Instant conditioner – A type of conditioner applied and left in the hair for about five minutes.

Invisible part weaves – A weave technique that involves making the weft, or tracks, look as though the extension hair is growing directly from the scalp.

Keratin – A threadlike protein, containing many compounds, that forms our hair and nails.

Lace front wig – A wig with a sheer attachment at the front that blends in with the hairline, giving the wig a more natural and believable look.

Leave-in conditioner – A type of conditioner that is left in the hair without rinsing out. Apply conditioner, comb through and then style as usual.

Medicated shampoo – Shampoo that treats the scalp and is formulated to assist dry and itchy scalp conditions, such as dandruff. Although impactful, it can be harsh on the hair.

Medulla – The innermost layer of the hair shaft.

Moisturizing conditioner – A type of conditioner that attracts moisture to the hair.

Moisturizing shampoo – A type of shampoo that contains humectants that attract moisture.

New growth – The natural Afro hair that grows from the scalp in the weeks after a chemical relaxer or a curly perm.

pH – A figure that describes the level of acidity or basicity in an aqueous or liquid solution.

Protective style – When Afro hair is styled, as opposed to kept loose, to prevent breakage and promote length retention. Styles include threading, cornrows, Bantu knots, twists outs, dreadlocks, etc.

Relaxing – A chemical process that changes the natural texture of Afro hair by breaking down its structure.

Remy hair – Human hair used for making contemporary wigs. Hair that has been chemically processed by the donor in the past.

Rod set – An alternative to curling the hair, without using curling tongs. Perm rods of various sizes can be used on natural, transitioning or relaxed hair.

Roller set – A method used to set long-lasting curls or to create waves. The size of the roller determines the tightness and size of the curl or wave.

Scalp – The skin on top of the human head, divided into three layers: the epidermis, dermis and subcutaneous layers.

Scarf – A fabric (usually silk) used to wrap natural hair at night to help retain moisture and prevent dryness and breakage. Often used instead of a silk pillowcase.

Sebaceous gland – A skin gland that secretes sebum into the hair follicles as a form of lubrication.

Sebum – Oil secreted from the sebaceous gland.

Sew in – A weave technique that involves cornrowing natural hair and sewing wefts into the rows.

Shampoo – A liquid product used to clean the hair.

Shrinkage – A decrease in length when hair goes from wet to dry.

Silk pillowcase – A covering for a pillow made of silk and used to retain moisture in the hair. Other fabrics, such as cotton, will dry hair out and will also break the hair whenever you toss and turn in your sleep.

Silk press – The use of a modern flat iron to straighten and press natural Afro hair.

Straw set – The use of drinking straws to set natural hair into coils.

Subcutaneous – The bottom layer of the skin.

Telogen – The last phase of the human hair growth cycle, also known as the resting phase, which lasts 100 days.

Tex-laxing – The use of a relaxer treatment to under-process the hair.

Threading – The process of wrapping wool, yarn or cotton thread evenly and unevenly around small sections of hair.

Traction alopecia – Bald patches caused by excessive manipulation and styling of the hair.

Transitioning – A process of growing out your natural hair texture before cutting off the processed or damaged ends from a relaxer.

Twist outs – A natural hairstyle involving two strand twists all over the head, which are then released to add texture to the hair.

Two strand twists – A protective style involving taking two strands of natural or synthetic hair and winding or twisting them tightly around each other until the very end.

Virgin hair – Human hair used for making contemporary wigs. Comes from a living person and a single donor and has not been processed by any chemical treatments such as dyes or perms.

Weave (or extensions) – Synthetic or human hair used to add length or fullness to natural hair, usually sewn in, clipped or glued.

Wig – A head covering made from human or synthetic hair. Many options exist for short, mid-length and longer styles. They can come in straight, wavy or curly textures and a variety of colours.

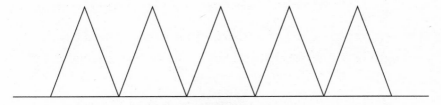

FAQS:
THE DOS AND DON'TS

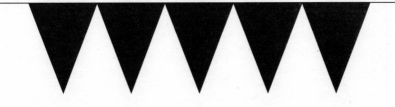

COMMON MISTAKES

Here are eight common mistakes made when caring for Afro hair, and how to solve them.

1. Damaging hair at night

If you don't wrap your hair before you go to bed, whilst you're asleep the pillow will absorb the moisture from your hair. This means that when you wake, your hair will appear dry, leading you to apply more products and heat to banish frizz.

Solution: Wrap hair with a silk scarf. This will help ensure the moisture is retained so you're less likely to need to resort to heated appliances and extra product, because your hair will already be beautifully hydrated.

2. Washing hair in hot water

Piping-hot water dries out the hair and strips away moisture.

Solution: Washing tresses in warm water will still cleanse effectively, plus it will help seal and be much gentler on the cuticle, resulting in a happier head of hair.

3. Not having regular treatments

Afro and curly textures can struggle in the cold weather. What's more, central heating can dry out the hair, leaving it dull and dehydrated.

Solution: It's so important to apply a treatment every two weeks to rehydrate, strengthen, protect and maintain hair health. A rich oil in-salon treatment such as my signature Manketti Treatment is ideal. After application at the backwash (sink), you'll be placed under a steamer for twenty minutes, as treatments work best when heat is applied. This helps to open the cuticle, enabling the nutrients to penetrate and nourish deeply within.

In between professional in-salon treatments, apply a masque to cleansed hair at home, or a small amount of butter, cream or pomade, to help transform frizzy hair into shinier tresses in as little as two minutes.

4. Blow-drying and ironing the hair too frequently

Blow-drying natural hair is all about the four Ts – treatment (using a moisturizing cream to protect hair), temperature control (keeping it low to medium), tension (not stretching or stressing wet hair) and technique (blow-drying in as little as five minutes). But constant blow-drying and ironing damages cuticles, splits the strands and dries out the hair.

Solution: Rather than blow-drying and tonging, try roller setting instead. As this involves less direct heat being applied to the hair, this option is a kinder way of getting hair smooth. And remember, whenever you're heat-styling your hair, always use protection first by applying a product to help guard against damage and leave hair shiny.

5. Not getting regular trims

As tempting as it may be to hold on to the length, it can do more harm than good. The ends of your hair are old and have been subjected to blow-drying, brushing, straightening, etc. so if you don't trim them, it won't style well. What's more, once the ends start to split, it travels up to mid-lengths, causing the damage to spread.

Solution: If you want your hair to style, curl and hold better, have trims every six weeks. Once the damaged hair is removed, it will look and feel so much healthier.

6. Not adding enough moisture

Afro and mixed-race hair needs regular moisture to be added – especially during the colder months.

Solution: Just as you moisturize your skin, try applying a good hydrating daily to prevent hair drying out. Don't overload the hair with product, though – just use a little bit more than you would during the summer. Two or three times a week apply a small amount of Manketti Oil and wrap hair in a silk scarf before bed for added hydration.

7. Having too many chemical treatments

Excessive use of chemical treatments can dry the hair, and incorrect application can cause damage.

Solution: Always have relaxers and colours applied professionally at a reputable salon. Rather than having six or seven relaxers throughout the year, try stretching out the frequency of application, for example, by having three or four but having steam treatments in between. This will help soften the regrowth, prevent breakage, plus strengthen.

8. Using the wrong hair bands

With the blustery weather conditions we endure for much of the year, it's tempting to quickly tie hair back, away from the wind and rain. However, using elastic or plastic bands will pull on the hair, resulting in damaged cuticles, friction and stress.

Solution: Use bands that are covered in either silk or satin. The smooth surface will help protect from breakage and damage, resulting in happier hair days, whatever the weather.

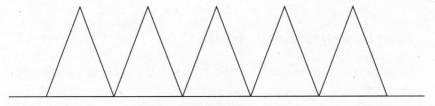

HOW TO:
HONE YOUR SKILLS

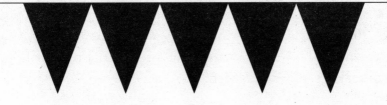

HOW TO: TREAT TRACTION ALOPECIA

As mentioned in Chapter 1, traction alopecia is a form of hair loss particularly around the hairline caused by excessive manipulation of the hair. Certain protective styles such as braiding can be damaging to the scalp due to excessively tight braids and overpulling, over a sustained period. Signs of traction alopecia include bumps and blisters, white pimples, itchiness, redness and soreness, and a generally tender scalp. Over time, if precautions are not taken, this will cause either temporary or permanent baldness around the hairline and other parts of the scalp.

Those who suffer from traction alopecia will have to be very patient when it comes to hair growth as it's not guaranteed that the hair will grow back at all once the hair follicle has been damaged. A consultation with a doctor is advised to see what's possible in terms of growth. If damage is not permanent, certain products specifically made for this type of hair loss can help to stimulate the hair follicle and promote growth, which can take up to a year to see any results. Certain products such as castor oil and hair supplements have a reputation for growing edges, but due to its thick consistency less is more, otherwise it will only clog up the pores. This option may suit some but not others, so experimentation with natural ingredients is key. A good massage and natural oil can help stimulate blood flow to affected areas in order to promote some growth. You may also want to speak with a doctor about medical treatments, if you feel this is right for you. The best advice is to keep the area clean with regular washing and to avoid any styles that require tight braiding, twisting and glue methods, which will serve to further irritate and clog the scalp.

HOW TO: GROW YOUR HAIR OUT

Although nutrition, hormones and genetics are the biggest determinants for length and thickness, here are five takeaway points to consider for optimal haircare and growth.

Moisturizing

Afro hair textures often become dry and brittle because the sebum produced by the scalp cannot reach the ends of the hair. The use of good-quality hair oils and butters helps to prevent breakage and keeps the hair hydrated. Shampoos and conditioners made to moisturize the hair are also integral to hair health, as are occasional deep treatments for added penetration. Don't forget the scalp while moisturizing, making sure to massage with one or two drops of oil to get the blood circulating and to penetrate the roots. I also recommend product cocktailing to accommodate all the different textures of the hair. You will need to experiment with a combination of gels, oils and mousses (and see how your hair responds) to create the perfect haircare regime for yourself.

Regular trims

Regular trims prevent split ends, which cause the hair to tangle, thin and break more easily. Hair that's trimmed will allow the hair to grow more readily. Women are often reluctant to have their hair trimmed because of length retention, but once the dead ends are removed, curls look and feel a whole lot better. Hair should always be trimmed by a professional in a reputable salon, otherwise you risk cutting off too much of your own hair, especially at the back, where it's difficult to see.

Minimal heat and chemical treatments

The use of heat and chemical treatments is automatically damaging to the hair, especially with repeated and frequent use. When possible, Afro hair should be dried naturally. If heat is required, try and use a low setting for blow-dryers and flat irons, and save this kind of drying for special occasions and salon visits. Chemical treatments such as relaxers should be avoided, especially for long-term haircare, and other ways of styling the hair should be considered in their place. Although colouring the hair provides a change in look or an option for covering grey hairs, colour treatments should be applied only occasionally, especially if you're thinking about the longevity and health of your hair.

Caution with protective styles

Although protective styles are important for length retention, for preventing excessive manipulation, and are excellent for the autumn and winter months, they can be harmful to the scalp if certain styles are applied with force or are kept in for too long. Our natural hair needs periods of rest from styling, and this includes looks that involve braiding, twisting and weave applications.

Night-time protection

Tossing and turning in the night creates dry and brittle hair, not to mention excessive tangling, especially if sleeping with cotton pillowcases, which suck moisture from the hair. In order to keep the hair hydrated, it's important to wrap your hair in a silk scarf before bed or to sleep with a silk pillowcase. I often suggest investing in a good scarf, which can be tied around the perimeter of the head, keeping the edges moisturized and smooth. Women with curlier curls can use the pineapple technique, gathering the hair up in the shape of the fruit and tying the scarf around the head.

HOW TO: CURL YOUR HAIR WITHOUT HEAT

Tips on adding definition

Generally speaking, twist outs or braids are the simplest way to add definition to your hair – and the bigger the braid or twist, the bigger the curl. Depending on your hair length, you can put the hair in anywhere from two to eight twists or braids and leave in for an hour or so (or until dry, if you've just washed your hair), with or without product, depending on your desired look. When you take out the twists and braids, you'll have beautiful waves or loose curls without having to do too much. You can also put the hair in rod sets or straw sets for more voluminous curls. However, there are plenty of ways to achieve natural curls.

- **Diffuser (hairdryer):** A diffuser is an accessory of the right size to fit your hairdryer. This is a great tool to use to even out your curl pattern(s). To give your curls some shape, simply turn your hairdryer on to the low setting and drop them into the diffuser. Scrunch the hair between your fingers. This will help maintain the curl formation.
- **Wash and go:** After you have shampooed and conditioned your hair, use curl enhancing products to add extra definition to your hair by reducing frizz. They also help it to stay in place for longer. Most of the curl enhancing products can be used on damp hair.
- **Finger coil:** This process involves using a great hydrating curl cream and your fingers to curl individual strands.
- **Comb twist:** Each twist is done by using a small toothcomb around small sections of hair. Start from the root and work your way down to the ends of the hair to create a drop curl.

- **Bantu knots:** Can be used to create some of the most defined curls – you can do anywhere between six and fifteen of these, depending on how big you want your curls to be, and this can take from forty-five minutes to two hours, depending on your hair length and volume. (They are best achieved on damp hair, as the moisture helps with the curl retention.) Feel free to keep them in for a few days before undoing the knots for super-defined curls.
- **Flexi rods:** Come in a range of different sizes, which will determine the size of your curls. Flexi rods form around hair with ease. Use on damp hair, leave them in overnight and pick them out in the morning for a head-turning do.
- **Rod (perm) sets:** Perm rods create the smoothest-looking curls. When done on damp hair, just let them dry completely.
- **Two strand twist:** One of the easiest methods for giving natural hair all-over curls comes from using two strand twists. Large sections of hair can be twisted into two strands around each other, then released for a full-wave pattern. For even more definition secure the ends with rods.
- **Flat twist:** More advanced than the two strand method. Flat twists are a technique that gives natural hair definition at the roots. Having parted hair in rows (like cornrows/canerows), twist those strands on to the scalp of

the head. This does take patience and practice and may be best achieved with the help of someone else.

- **Braid-out:** A braid-out is perhaps the most straightforward way to achieve a fresh look, and can be done one of two ways: using individual plaits or cornrows. Either way, you will end up with a defined Z-shaped pattern.
- **Straw set:** This gives a similar feel to flexi rods. Use your spare plastic or paper straws and wrap small sections of hair in an upward motion, finishing at the root of the hair. Secure the hair and straw together with a hairpin.
- **Curlformers:** Curlformers come in a variety of lengths and sizes but are often soft and colourful corkscrew-shaped hair curlers. You simply clip your strands around the inner hook and pull through. You can sleep in them overnight, and will enjoy a smooth, looser curl as the beautiful end result.

HOW TO: STRAIGHTEN HAIR WITHOUT HEAT

We explored threading in Chapter 2, but there are several techniques to use for straighter hair, which do not require any heat. Here are a few of them.

- **African threading:** It's a great method for both stretching and straightening natural hair. Part your hair into sections and wrap the thread around each section.

205

- **Hair wrap:** Wrap damp hair by brushing flat against your head. After wrapping smooth, use a silk scarf to cover the head. Allow four to six hours, depending on the length of hair. When the time is up, you will reveal a sleek, straight head of hair.
- **Roller set:** Roller sets have multiple uses – you can also use rollers to straighten your hair. When your hair is damp, apply your favourite setting products and then start rolling. Remember to ensure a consistent tension throughout, so your straightening results are nice and even.

HOW TO: FIND THE RIGHT HAIRSTYLE FOR YOU

The most common mistake most people make when trying to determine their face shape is thinking that their face is simply round. When determining your face shape, you should be looking at your hairline, width and length of your face, and also your jaw-line. The easiest way to know what face shape you have is to pull your hair back, take an eyeliner, look in the mirror and trace the outline of your face.

Your face shape should fall within one of the following categories: oval face, square face, round face, heart-shaped face, long face or diamond face. There are hairstyles that suit each face shape, but also styles to avoid, as in the table below.

Oval face	Best styles	Hairstyles to avoid
Length of face is longer than width. Jawline is slightly narrower than hairline	Works well with all hairstyles. Sleek hairstyles, blunt bobs, pixies, tapered cuts	One-length styles (keep them from dragging the face down)
Square face	Best styles	Hairstyles to avoid
Strong angled jawline. Forehead, cheekbones and jawline are the same width	Layered bobs, graduated tapered cuts, short bobs, blunt fringes, waves and curls	Styles that draw too much attention to the jawline (high buns, etc.)
Round face	Best styles	Hairstyles to avoid
Width and length are the same, also known as 'baby face'	Deep side part, high ponytail, tapered cuts with volume on top	One-length cuts and full curls, which can balloon the face
Heart-shaped face	Best styles	Hairstyles to avoid
Hairline is the widest part of the face. Narrow chin and prominent cheekbones	Shoulder-length, deep side part with loose waves, space buns	Middle parting and short fringes

Long face	Best styles	Hairstyles to avoid
Similar to oval face, with a long chin	Blow-out with volume, loose curls and waves	Very long hair, sleek hairstyles
Diamond face	Best styles	Hairstyles to avoid
Forehead and jawline are the same width. Cheekbones are the widest part of the face	Short textured bob, sleek high ponytail	Heavy fringes

HOW TO: AVOID FRIZZ

Humidity, heat and a lack of moisture are all contributors to a frizzy head of hair. In order to combat this, moisturizing is essential. When washing the hair, use moisturizing shampoos containing extra emollients. Always condition the hair and use deep treatments when necessary, and continually oil the hair or use butters. Keratin treatments (as mentioned in Chapter 3) can also provide a temporary solution for frizz-free hair. Protective styles are also a sure way to avoid dealing with frizz, as your hair is hidden from the elements and tucked away.

HOW TO: PROTECT YOUR HAIR WHEN EXERCISING/SWIMMING

When swimming in chlorinated water, it's best to wet your locks prior to entering the pool. Wet hair is less absorbent than dry hair, so wetting the hair beforehand reduces the chances of hair taking in the damaging effects of chlorine, such as discoloration and dryness. The same technique can be used when swimming in the ocean or sea, where hair will be more prone to dryness. You can also add a layer of conditioner to the hair to act as a protective barrier. Hair should always be shampooed, conditioned and oiled after swimming to clean the hair and replenish moisture.

Afro hair can become frizzy while exercising, due to heat and perspiration. Depending on your workout routine, and how often you choose to go to the gym, hair should be washed a little more frequently to remove product build-up and sweat – but not too much, otherwise moisture and oils are stripped from the hair and scalp. Hair should be tied up and kept away from the face while exercising. Use protective styles, such as cornrows, braids and twists, to avoid touching the hair too much or battling with frizz. (If you can, and your style calls for it, try getting your hands on a dreadlocks swim cap online – this works wonders with heavier styles.)

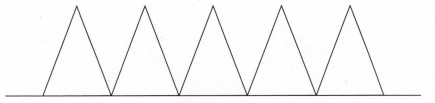

HOW TO:
FIND YOUR HAIR ESSENTIALS

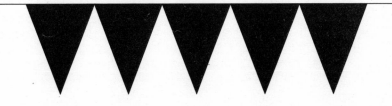

WHAT TO BUY

So, you've made it to the shop. But now what should you put in your basket? What are the essentials that will help you maintain your hair? Below, I outline the utensils that every person with Afro, curly or otherwise textured hair should have for the maintenance of healthy and happy hair, as well as some of my go-to products.

Your shopping list

- **Tail combs** – used for precise parting and for sculpturing baby hairs.
- **Wide toothcomb** – used to separate and detangle damp and wet hair after applying conditioner or detangling lotion.
- **Afro combs** – used to pick out Afros or to loosen hair completely. They can also be used to style various looks, such as the twist out, for extra lift.
- **Paddle brush** – used for detangling the hair and to eliminate knots. Also used for blow-drying, wrapping the hair and massaging the scalp.
- **Butterfly clips** – used to hold large sections of already-separated textured hair, as well as locs.
- **Hairpins** – large and small hairpins are used for styling all textures.

- **Spray bottle** – detangling your hair without any water can cause breakage. Use a mixture of water and conditioner to loosen up any knots before shampooing.
- **Silk scarves** – help to retain the moisture and natural oils in your hair. They don't absorb moisture out of your hair like cotton and synthetic materials.
- **Silk pillowcase** – helps to retain the natural oils in your hair.
- **Headwrap** – perfect for days when your twist-out/braids won't cooperate or when you want to try something a little different.
- **Moisturizing shampoos** – contain humectants that attract moisture. Some of my favourites are Manketti Oil shampoo, Afrocenchix, Big Hair + beauty, Jim + Henry.
- **Conditioning shampoos** – used to treat dry, brittle and damaged hair, as well as chemically treated and colour-processed hair. If you can stretch, try Manketti Oil shampoo, Briogeo, Dizziak, Afrocenchix.
- **Leave-in conditioners** – should be used after normal shampoo and conditioner. Try Shea Moisture, Cantu, Briogeo, Philip Kingsley.
- **Moisturizing conditioners** – attract moisture to the hair. I recommend Manketti Oil conditioner, Afrocenchix, KeraCare Humecto, Briogeo.
- **Deep penetrating conditioners** – should be used once a month or every two weeks, depending on the condition of the hair, especially after braids and hair extensions are removed.

- **Shea butter** – can be used as a moisturizer, conditioner and healing agent for the scalp. Natural shea butter is imported and can be bought online or in hair shops and is usually quite affordable.
- **Exfoliating treatments** – salt scrubs work to remove dead skin cells and excess sebum that can block hair follicles. They also help with the blood circulation, promoting smoother and healthier hair growth.
- **Essential oils** – oils that are rich in fatty acids and vitamin E help to hydrate dry, coarse, unruly hair, creating softer and shinier, more manageable hair, whilst cutting out frizz and flyaways, too.
- **Finishing products** – used sparingly and only after hair has been styled.
- **Gels** – some good gels include Aunt Jackie's Flaxseed Gel, Curlsmith curl defining styling soufflé, Shea Moisture coconut enhancing smoothie.
- **Mousse** – best applied to wet hair to set and redefine the curl pattern. Try Paul Mitchell, Shea Moisture or Design Essentials.
- **Edge control** – to help smooth out flyaways or baby hairs.
- **Hairspray** – for sheen and to hold your hair in place.
- **Curl creme** – this will moisturize your hair and give your curls more definition. Check out the Bouclème and Aveda Be Curly ranges.
- **Pomades** – Aveda brilliant humectant pomade, Mizani rose H_2O conditioning hairdress or Manketti Oil pomade.

- **Blow-dryer** – a beauty essential. There is a blow-dryer for every purse, but if you can invest, try Dyson or GHD.
- **Diffuser** – bowl-shaped attachment that disperses the flow of air from your blow-dryer, helping to dry your curls more evenly and gently, whilst preventing frizz, encouraging definition and creating volume.
- **Afropik** – a hairdryer accessory that is ideal for blow-drying Afro and curly textures as the pik attachment allows hot air to be distributed throughout your hair.

READING THE SMALL PRINT

Another thing many people tell me when they come to my salon is how confusing language on products can be. Labels often look different to one another but on closer inspection they contain similar information, and much of it is often shared as a legal requirement. Some of the common information you will find includes: *brand name and product name; product type/purpose; ingredients list; symbols; usage/directions/weight*. The order of the ingredients listed on the label is important. Ingredients are listed in descending order, from the greatest amount to the least amount present in the product.

Understanding hair product labels

I've put together this list so that you can feel empowered while shopping for your hair products and know exactly what's going on to your head.

- **Parabens:** also known as **butylparaben**, **methylparaben** and (more commonly) **propylparaben**, these are synthetic chemicals that are used as preservatives in a variety of products including hair products. Parabens are derived from a chemical known as para-hydroxybenzoic acid (PHBA) that occurs naturally in many fruits and vegetables, such as blueberries and carrots.
- **Silicone:** often used in shampoo, conditioners and styling products to help create the slip needed to detangle and give hair a silky shine. Silicone is also used as a heat protectant.
- **Water:** acts as a solvent, keeping the other ingredients in solution.
- **Ammonium laureth sulfate** and **ammonium lauryl sulfate:** detergents that remove oils and grease from hair.
- **Dimethicone:** a conditioning ingredient that makes dry hair soft.
- **Glycol distearate:** gives shampoo a pearlescent look.
- **Cocamide MEA:** a lather builder.
- **Hydrolysed collagen** and **tricetylmonium chloride:** conditioning ingredients that help control static and make hair easier to comb.
- **Stearyl alcohol:** fatty alcohol, used in shampoos and conditioners so that the product can spread through the hair better.
- **Methylisothiazolinone:** fragrance.

FINDING 'GOOD' HAIR PRODUCTS

Now that you know what each ingredient does, the question is, how do you know what makes a good product?

Shampoo

A good shampoo should clean away oil and dirt, rinse out easily and leave your hair shiny and manageable. To get oil and build-up out of your hair, you need detergent. Using detergent on your hair sounds a little harsh, but I can tell you it's a good idea. Washing your hair with water alone doesn't get out the build-up and oil.

Conditioner

A good conditioner leaves a smooth waxy coating on the hair, strengthening the cuticle or forming a protective layer over the cortex where cuticle cells have broken away. Hair can become tangled when the lifted edges of the cuticle layer on one hair get caught on the cuticle layer of another hair. By adding coating that smooths out these rough edges, conditioner helps keep your hair from tangling.

Oils

A good hair oil is meant to replicate and supplement the oils that our bodies already make. Hair oils smell nice and provide you with control over the amount and application.

Serums

A good serum will help protect your hair against the sun's harmful rays. Serums containing hydrating oils like jojoba, argan or sweet almond oils make curly hair more manageable and frizz-free.

HOW TO CREATE YOUR OWN HAIR PRODUCTS

Many home ingredients are also rich in fatty acids, vitamins and minerals. Many serve as natural **emollients** (a cream or liquid that soothes and softens the skin) or **humectants** (a substance that maintains or seals in moisture) or contain antifungal and antibacterial properties which are good for dry and itchy scalps. Some home ingredients may assist in hair growth or help prevent hair loss.

Foods rich in nutrients are not only good for dietary health, which is very important to hair vitality and growth, but can also be applied to the hair as masks and deep conditioning treatments.

Egg yolks, for example, are high in protein and packed with vitamins A, D and E. They are often thought to strengthen the hair and prevent breakage, although this may not work for everyone. A good-quality honey is known to have antioxidant, antifungal and antibacterial properties, all of which help hair conditions like dandruff (depending on the severity). Honey also serves as a natural emollient and humectant, making it great for combating dry and frizzy hair.

Avocados are another superfood, often hailed for health and used in hair masks. They are high in monounsaturated fatty acids and have loads of vitamins. Below are a few of my favourite recipes to try at home. They work as masks and will act as a deep moisturizing treatment for dry and brittle hair.

TIPS & TRICKS

Deep conditioning recipe #1: Egg yolk mask

Blend the following ingredients together in a bowl to form a smooth paste.

- 2 tablespoons of honey
- 2 tablespoons of olive oil

- 2 tablespoons of lemon juice
- 2 egg yolks

Step by step

1. Shampoo the hair as normal and towel dry, leaving the hair slightly damp.
2. Apply the mixture evenly throughout the hair and comb through with a wide toothcomb for even distribution.
3. Leave on for fifteen minutes.
4. When the time is up, rinse off thoroughly,
5. Apply a conditioner and leave it on for five minutes, then rinse it out.
6. Dry and style as usual.

Deep conditioning recipe #2: Shea butter and avocado mask

Shea butter is a conditioner, moisturiser and healing agent for the scalp. It's made from the West African shea nut and is excellent for controlling hair loss. Shea butter works well on Afro/curly hair types, tames frizz, reduces split ends, protects damaged hair and hydrates hair.

Time: 30 minutes

- 1 tablespoon of shea butter
- 2 tablespoons of coconut oil
- 1 teaspoon of Manketti Oil
- Half an avocado

Step by step

1. Heat the coconut oil and shea butter together until it makes a runny mixture.
2. Add the Manketti Oil and avocado then whip all the ingredients until they are smooth.
3. Section the hair into four parts applying the mixture to the hair, working it into the roots and down to the ends.
4. Once the hair is fully covered, let the mask sit for about 30 minutes.
5. Proceed to wash hair with cool water and mild home-made shampoo.

Deep conditioning recipe #3: Coconut oil mask

Blend the following ingredients together in a bowl to form a smooth paste.

- 2 tablespoons of coconut oil
- 2 tablespoons of cinnamon (known to stimulate blood circulation and promote hair growth)

Step by step

1. Shampoo the hair as normal and towel dry, leaving the hair slightly damp.
2. Massage the paste evenly throughout the hair, from the roots down to the ends.
3. Leave on for thirty minutes.
4. Rinse, condition and style as usual.

Natural reconstructive masque

Mix the following ingredients together in a small bowl until they are thoroughly blended.

- Half a cup of honey
- 3 teaspoons of olive oil
- 1 tablespoon of guar gum
- 4 drops of essential rosemary oil

Step by step

1. Apply the mixture to damp hair, making sure to coat the hair completely.
2. Cover hair with a plastic cap for about thirty minutes.
3. Shampoo lightly.
4. Rinse thoroughly with cool water to remove the conditioner, before styling.

Leave-in conditioner

Follow these steps to add moisture and sheen to your hair before styling. Blend the following ingredients in a spray bottle.

- 4 cups of warm water
- A quarter of a cup of fresh lemon juice
- 2 teaspoons of pure honey

Step by step

1. Mix all the ingredients thoroughly.
2. Spray the mixture on to freshly washed hair.

Scalp invigorator

This is a stimulating antiseptic for an itchy scalp.

- 2 tablespoons of rosemary oil
- 1 tablespoon of jojoba oil
- 1 tablespoon of iodine

Step by step

1. Combine ingredients and massage into the scalp for ten minutes.
2. Leave in. Do not rinse.
3. Do this twice a week to relieve an itchy, tight scalp.

Moisturizing cleanser

Mix the following ingredients thoroughly in a small bowl.

- 2 tablespoons of Epsom salt
- 2 tablespoons of baking soda
- 2 tablespoons of aloe vera gel
- 2 tablespoons of apple cider vinegar
- 2 tablespoons of chamomile tea
- A quarter of a cup of vegetable-based liquid soap

Step by step

1. Shampoo hair twice.
2. Condition and style as usual.
3. This will leave the hair soft and shiny.

Natural shampoo

Combine the following ingredients in a bottle and shake well until thoroughly blended.

- A quarter of a cup of warm water
- A quarter of a cup of organic liquid vegetable-based soap
- Half a teaspoon of organic oil (for example, sunflower oil or olive oil)

Step by step

1. Use this mixture to shampoo your hair twice.
2. Apply conditioner.
3. Style hair as usual.

Apple cider shampoo

Apple cider vinegar is great as a natural rinse out. It not only makes your hair smoother, but it also makes it easier to detangle, meaning less breakage.

Time: 5 minutes

- 2 tablespoons baking soda
- 2 cups water
- 3 tablespoons apple cider vinegar
- 1 teaspoon of Charlotte Mensah Manketti Hair Oil

STYLING IT OUT: COMBS AND BRUSHES

You want to style your hair – but what should you use to do so? Below is a list of combs and brushes and each of their uses.

Paddle brush

Paddle brushes come in a variety of sizes, depending on how long or thick your hair is. They are good for all hair types and are primarily used for detangling wet or dry hair and preventing split ends. Not all paddle brushes are made for Afro and curly hair textures so look for ones that detangle the hair gently, otherwise they will cause damage from unnecessary tugging and pulling. A good paddle brush massages the scalp, stimulating blood flow and polishing the cuticles in the process. It's best to opt for brushes made of materials that are heat resistant and easy to wash and air-dry. Use a brush without knots on the bristles if you can.

Round brush

Round brushes are mostly used for styling. They're a great tool for blow-drying longer hair textures for a smooth and silky finish. Round brushes have bristles distributed all around a barrel. The shape allows for a continuous straightening or curling movement during the drying process, which creates lots of body and bounce. Hair becomes less frizzy, as the barrel of the brush is usually made with a metal base. The brush comes in a variety of sizes, depending on your desired look.

Afro comb (or Pik)

Afro combs or Piks are a wonderful tool to use for more volume on Afro hair or certain protective styles such as **twist outs**. These combs make hair look fuller by raising kinks and coils. They are used primarily for styling but can also be used to loosen hair before trimming. When picking, always comb Afro hair from the roots and lift gently upwards, removing the Pik around mid-length or when the comb sticks. Never try and force the comb through to the ends as this will damage the hair, causing breakage. Piks are vertical in shape with a handle at the top to grip while picking. They are usually made from plastic, metal or even wood, and have long teeth.

Wide toothcomb

Wide toothcombs are good tools for combing Afro hair, especially when detangling or distributing conditioner or products throughout the hair. The general rule of thumb is the wider the teeth, the better for thicker hair textures, as the teeth will be able to glide through the hair more easily. Use combs when the hair is wet for curly and Afro hair textures, and with the use of products, for easier management. Wide toothcombs come in all shapes and sizes, depending on hair texture and length.

Tail combs

Tail combs are a great styling implement and have two primary functions. They have tools on either end to both comb and section the hair. The teeth on the comb are very fine, making it useful for teasing the hair for additional volume. The comb is also good for slicking down edges and baby hairs, especially with products like pomades and butters. The sectioning tool creates very precise partings and is often good for dividing the hair when braiding or cornrowing.

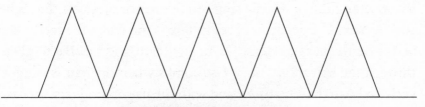

YOUR HAIR HEALTH: CHARTING YOUR HAIR

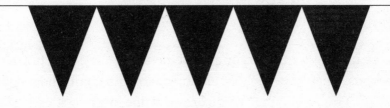

YOUR HAIR HEALTH THROUGHOUT THE SEASONS

What is your ultimate hair goal – hair growth, more volume, regrowing your hairline, transitioning? Regardless of what you wish to do, it's easier to achieve if you're making notes. Just like we devise different skin regimes, our hair necessitates special care during different times of the year in order to thrive. Sporting a range of hairstyles throughout the year can not only be a good way of giving your hair a break from certain potentially damaging styles, it can also be really good in terms of promoting hair growth, as well as a fun thing to do. Clients often ask me when they should be looking to try out new hairdos, so here is an outline of the best way to keep your hair healthy during different seasons (this advice will, of course, vary depending on where in the world you live).

Autumn and winter

Cold weather climates and dry air can be brutal for Afro and curly hair textures, which is why it's a good idea to keep hair in protective styles and to increase the use of oils and rich butters for extra moisture. Protective styles help to retain moisture and keep your natural hair away from the elements. The use of heavier oils and butters will also help to replenish your locks.

Good protective styles for the winter include: **weaves**, **corn-rows**, **Bantu knots** and **braids**.

Spring and summer

During the summer months, it's easy for Afro hair to become dehydrated and frizzy due to heat and humidity, which can cause additional breakage. The best way to combat this is to regularly deep-condition the hair, drink plenty of water and, of course, continue with your haircare regime, such as sleeping with your silk scarf to further retain moisture. Try and keep shampooing to a minimum and use moisturizing shampoos containing extra emollients or products formulated for dry hair. For women with curlier hair textures, diffuse your curls on a low heat and refrain from touching the hair too much. This is a good time to rock natural hair or to leave the hair out, but make sure to keep the hair hydrated at all times.

Good protective styles for the spring and summer include: **twist outs** and **spiral rod sets**.

YOUR HAIR HEALTH CHART: WEEKLY

I recommend you track your hair health and routine over the course of a week, using a chart such as the one here. Repeat for every week of the month.

	Dryness	Brittleness	Shampoo	Conditioning	Deep Conditioning	Oil (list type)	Heat
Monday							
Tuesday							
Wednesday							
Thursday							
Friday							
Saturday							
Sunday							

Notes:

_____

_____

_____

_____

_____

_____

_____

_____

YOUR HAIR HEALTH CHART: ONE YEAR

How does your hair health vary throughout the year? Fill in this hair health diary to chart your hair progress. This is a really good way of figuring out which styles best suit your lifestyle.

	Season	Length	Dryness	Texture	Style	Weather	Location	Comments
Week 1								
Week 2								
Week 3								
Week 4								
Week 5								
Week 6								
Week 7								
Week 8								
Week 9								
Week 10								
Week 11								
Week 12								
Week 13								
Week 14								

	Season	Length	Dryness	Texture	Style	Weather	Location	Comments
Week 15								
Week 16								
Week 17								
Week 18								
Week 19								
Week 20								
Week 21								
Week 22								
Week 23								
Week 24								
Week 25								
Week 26								
Week 27								
Week 28								
Week 29								
Week 30								
Week 31								
Week 32								
Week 33								

	Season	Length	Dryness	Texture	Style	Weather	Location	Comments
Week 34								
Week 35								
Week 36								
Week 37								
Week 38								
Week 39								
Week 40								
Week 41								
Week 42								
Week 43								
Week 44								
Week 45								
Week 46								
Week 47								
Week 48								
Week 49								
Week 50								
Week 51								
Week 52								

Notes:

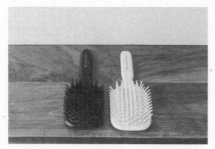

Paddle brushes, black and white

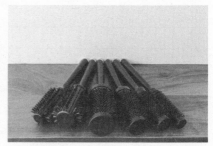

Round brushes

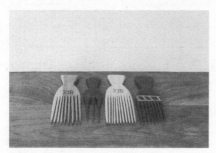

Afro comb and Afro Pik

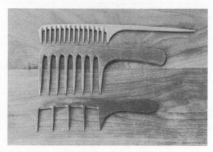

Wide toothcomb

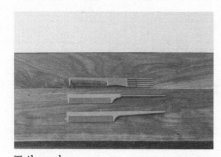

Tail comb

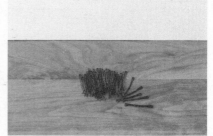

Hair pins

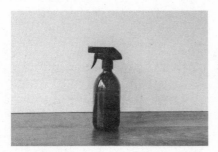

Spray bottle

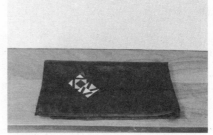

Silk scarf

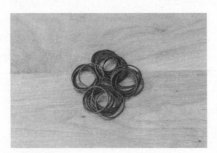

Hair bands

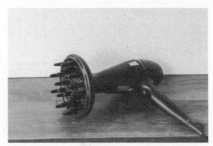

Diffuser on blowdryer

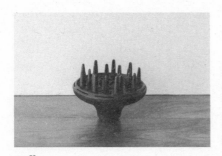

Diffuser

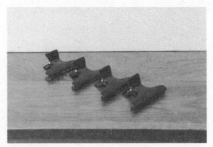

Butterfly clips

AFTERWORD

THE YEAR OF RETURN AND THE FUTURE OF AFRO HAIR

Growth is the plan for the future – both that of my haircare brand and my own growth.

The Manketti Oil Haircare range is really a way of projecting my work across the world, and that requires me being in more places. The range is now stocked by beauty and fashion outlets such as Space NK & Net-a-Porter, who ship globally. If the products are everywhere, I too need to be everywhere. Making the brand accessible is one thing, but building a community takes a lot more time and has a lot more lasting effect on success. We're currently seeing orders coming through from East Asia to South Africa, so creating a regional presence has to be the next step.

In terms of my own personal development, I feel like playing a more active role in the hair and beauty industry on an executive level. I've become a board member of the British Beauty Council and the Institute for Apprenticeships and Technical Education, helping the latter in building up their offering for hairdressing apprenticeships with a specific focus on Afro and curly hair types. Along with both these positions I'm also an ambassador for The

Prince's Trust, which goes hand in hand with Love Naa Densua, a project which, going forward, I intend to build out further, both in the UK and in Ghana.

As a global authority on textured hair, I believe it will be a lot more of the same. I've consulted for a number of prestigious global brands like L'Oréal & GHD as well as providing hair direction on shoots with the world's biggest publications.

In terms of trends, I don't think Afro or curly hair types are one; we have consistently been adventurous, innovative and trail-blazing with the many ways in which we wear our hair. Now we're just more visible in the mainstream media, and there's a very clear benefit to that.

I think it's great – the widespread embrace we're seeing of natural hair. I was in New York last summer, and I was loving all the natural hairstyles I saw on women with curly hair textures. Afros, TWAs, buzz cuts, twist outs, braids, dreadlocks – I saw it all. I even look at my son, who's transitioned from having a buzz cut to growing his hair and twisting it. I'm in the process of growing out my natural hair, using braids as a protective style; I'm super-excited to see the growth and all the cool things I can do with it.

I think there's a trend of people feeling empowered to be themselves, and not letting anything hold them back in that, be it family, friends or even working environment. I champion this and encourage people to be comfortable in themselves; wear a weave if you like, wear your hair natural if that's what you prefer.

But above all, do it for yourself.

FURTHER READING AND RESOURCES

Books

Bones, Jah, *One Love: History, Doctrine & Livity*, Voice of Rasta Publishing House, 1985.

Boone, Sylvia Ardyn, *Radiance from the Waters: Ideals of Feminine Beauty in Mende Art*, Yale University Press, 1986.

Byrd, Ayana D. and Tharps, Lori L., *Hair Story: Untangling the Roots of Black Hair in America*, St Martin's Press, 2001.

Carey, Alexander Timothy, *Colonial Students: A Study of the Social Adaptation of Colonial Students in London*, Secker & Warburg, 1956.

Fisher, Angela, *Africa Adorned*, William Collins, 1984.

Gundara, Jagdish S. and Duffield, Ian (eds), *Essays on the History of Blacks in Britain*, Avebury, 1992.

Hatton, Lesley and Hatton, Phillip, *Perming and Straightening: A Salon Handbook* (Second Edition), Blackwell Scientific Publications, 1993.

Hatton, L., Hatton, P. and Powell, A., *Colouring: A Salon Handbook*, Collins Professional and Technical Books, 1986.

Hatton, Phillip, *Afro Hair: A Salon Handbook*, Blackwell Scientific Publications, 1994.

Hausner, Sondra L., *Wandering with Sadhus: Ascetics in the Hindu Himalayas*, Indiana University Press, 2007.

Jell-Bahlsen, Sabine, *Mammy Water in Igbo Culture*, EZU Books, 2014.

McKissack, Patricia and McKissack, Fredrick, *Madam C. J. Walker: Self-Made Millionaire*, Enslow, 1992.

Mastalia, Francesco and Pagano, Alfonse, *Dreads*, Artisan, 1999.

National Research Council, *Lost Crops of Africa: Volume II: Vegetables*, National Academies Press, 2006, Chapter 17 'Shea', pp. 302–21.

Phillips, Mike and Phillips, Trevor, *Windrush: The Irresistible Rise of Multi-Racial Britain*, HarperCollins, 1998.

Roberti, Amanda and Hetfield, Lisa, 'Madam C. J. Walker: Leadership Grounded in Social and Racial Uplift' in Lisa Hetfield and Dana M. Britton (eds), *Junctures in Women's Leadership: Business*, Rutgers University Press, 2016.

Scobie, Edward, *Black Britannia: A History of Blacks in Britain*, Johnson Publishing, 1972.

Sherrow, Victoria, *Encyclopedia of Hair: A Cultural History*, Greenwood Press, 2006.

Smith, M. G., Augier, R. and Nettleford, R., *The Ras Tafari Movement in Kingston, Jamaica*, University College of the West Indies Institute of Social and Economic Research, 1960.

Swift, Alan J., *Fundamentals of Human Hair Science*, Micelle Press, 1997.

Magazines and newspapers

'Awareness Around Hair Bias', *Little Black Book*, 14 September 2018.

Black Voices, 'New York City Aims to Stop Hair Discrimination', *Huffington Post*, 18 February 2019.

Byrd, Ayana and Tharps, Lori L., 'When Black Hair is Against the Rules', *The New York Times*, 30 April 2014.

Davies, Caroline, 'London school that told boy to cut off dreadlocks backs down', *The Guardian*, 12 September 2018.

Driver, George, 'What is Balayage? Everything You Need to Know About the A-List Hair Technique', *Elle*, 8 November 2019.

Frazer-Carroll, Micha, 'Young Black Brits on Growing up with Hair Discrimination: "It Stays with You"', *Huffington Post*, 5 March 2019.

Garside, Jen and Winter, Lottie, 'I tried the keratin hair treatment Meghan Markle swears by for sleek, glossy ends and it changed my life', *Glamour Magazine*, 26 April 2019.

Muttucumaru, Ayesha, 'Not Fair: Literally Everything You Need to Know About Hair Weaves', *Get the Gloss*, 9 August 2017.

Phillips, Caryl, 'The Real Meaning of "Rachmanism"', *The New York Review of Books*, 23 December 2019.

Pometsey, Olive, 'Charlotte Mensah's 6 Tips For Achieving the Natural Hair of Your Dreams', *Elle*, 14 June 2018.

Pometsey, Olive, 'Just a Super Useful Guide to Getting Faux Locs', *Elle*, 15 June 2018.

Princess Gabbara, 'Cornrows and Sisterlocks and Their Long History', *Ebony Magazine*, 20 January 2017.

Princess Gabbara, 'Everything You Need to Know About Bantu Knots', *Ebony Magazine*, 29 November 2016.

Proudfoot, Jenny, 'Here's everything you need to know about getting a Keratin hair treatment', *Marie Claire*, 17 October 2017.

Rhule, Shevelle, 'Are You Ready to Tex-Lax?' *Pride Magazine*, 14 December 2015.

Richards, Kimberley, 'Video of High School Wrestler Forced to Cut Locs Sparks Outrage', *Huffington Post*, 21 December 2018.

Richards, Merissa, 'Black Londoner Teaches Bulgarians How to Style Afro Hair', *The Voice*, 2 July 2011.

Rosenstein, Jenna, '8 Things to Know About Hair-Smoothing Keratin Treatments', *Allure*, 7 December 2017.

'The one thing that may give away when Meghan Markle is pregnant', *Cosmopolitan*, 31 August 2018.

Turner, Elle, 'I tried hair steaming and it transformed my hair. Here's everything you need to know . . .' *Glamour Magazine*, 30 October 2019.

Whitbread, Louise, 'How Not to End Up With a Sh*t Haircut – We Asked the Experts', *Huffington Post*, 8 November 2019.

White, Nadine, 'Lessons Learned in 2018: Schools Must Do More to Foster Diversity and Inclusion', *Huffington Post*, 29 December 2018.

Woo, Elaine, 'Comer Cottrell dies at 82; made Jheri Curl available to the masses', *Los Angeles Times*, 8 October 2014.

Yedroudj, Latifa, 'Meghan Markle baby: The ONE CLUE that could reveal when Meghan becomes pregnant', *Daily Express*, 3 October 2018.

Young, Sarah, 'The Ultimate Summer Haircare Routine for Afro-Textured and Curly Hair', *The Independent*, 21 June 2019.

Journals

Elias, Marlène and Carney, Judith, 2007, 'African Shea Butter: A Feminized Subsidy from Nature', *AFRICA: Journal of the International African Institute*, 77 (1), 37: https://doi.org/10.3366/afr.2007.77.1.37

Fletcher, J. and Salamone, F., 2016, 'An Ancient Egyptian Wig: Construction and Reconstruction', *Internet Archaeology*, 42: http://dx.doi.org/10.11141/ia.42.6.3

Joseph-Salisbury, Remi and Connelly, Laura, 2018, ' "If Your Hair Is Relaxed, White People Are Relaxed. If Your Hair Is Nappy, They're Not Happy": Black Hair as a Site of "Post-Racial" Social Control in English Schools', *Social Sciences*, 7(11), 219: https://doi.org/10.3390/socsci7110219

Pratt, C., King, L., Messenger, A. et al., 2017, 'Alopecia Areata', *Nature Reviews Disease Primers*, 3, 17011: https://doi.org/10.1038/nrdp.2017.11

Online resources

American Shea Butter Institute, '21 Reasons to Use Shea Butter', 2013: https://www.sheainstitute.com/asbi-library/21reasons/

Ashton, Sally-Ann, 'Origins of the Afro Comb: 6000 years of culture, politics and identity', The Fitzwilliam Museum, 2013: http://maa.cam.ac.uk/origins-of-the-afro-comb-6000-years-of-culture-politics-and-identity/

British Foundation, 'Alopecia Areata: What is alopecia areata?': https://www.britishskinfoundation.org.uk/alopecia-areata

Calder, J. and Macfarlane, B., 'How are Ethnic Hairstyles Really Viewed in the Workplace?' 2016, retrieved December 2019 from Cornell University, ILR School site: http://digitalcommons.ilr.cornell.edu/student/139

Donnelly, Sue, 'Kwame Nkrumah (1909–1972) – a term at LSE', 10 October 2018: https://blogs.lse.ac.uk/lsehistory/2018/10/10/kwame-nkrumah-lse/

Gregory, Phil, 'Black British Timeline', Black Presence in Britain website, 15 September 2009: https://blackpresence.co.uk/black-british-timeline/

Griffin, Chanté, 'How Natural Black Hair at Work Became a Civil Rights Issue', JSTOR DAILY, 3 July 2019: https://daily.jstor.org/how-natural-black-hair-at-work-became-a-civil-rights-issue/

'History of Cornrow Braiding': https://csdt.org/culture/legacy/african/CORNROW_CURVES/culture/african.origins.htm

'How Can Shea Butter Be Used on My Skin and Hair?',
Healthline Media: https://www.healthline.com/health/
shea-butter-for-hair

Lemelson-MIT Program, 'Jheri Redding': http://lemelson.mit.
edu/resources/jheri-redding

Mintel Press Office, 'Natural Hair Movement Drives Sales of
Styling Products in US Black Haircare Market', 17 December
2015: https://www.mintel.com/press-centre/beauty-and-
personal-care/natural-hair-movement-drives-sales-of-styling-
products-in-us-black-haircare-market

'Music hairstyles: a brief history of 12 iconic cuts', BBC,
14 October 2016: https://www.bbc.co.uk/music/articles/
0125caa8-a00d-4bf8-98e1-089e2dac254f

Newport Jr, Jean Paul, 'The King of Shampoo: Jheri Redding's
latest company is aiming at beauty salons', CNN, 2 September
1985: https://money.cnn.com/magazines/fortune/fortune_
archive/1985/09/02/66389/index.htm

Sini, Rozina, 'Wear a weave at work – your afro hair is
unprofessional', BBC, 15 May 2016: https://www.bbc.co.uk/
news/uk-36279845

ACKNOWLEDGEMENTS

To God I give all the praise and glory, it's through you I feel empowered to achieve all things. It was written.

To my late brother, Ferdinand Kusi Thompson. A shining light of positivity whom we all miss dearly. A man who would give you the clothes off his back and saw the optimism in every situation. I love you and thank you for all your help along the years.

Bashiru, thank you for a consistent source of support, from helping in the salon to proofreading this book! You're the best son I could wish for and I'm immensely proud of you.

To my late Mum, Grandma and Grandpa for instilling and creating my life, I channel your energies into everything I do. The legacy continues.

To my amazing Father for teaching me the value of hard work, and the fact that it's the cornerstone for everything.

Babs, words can never be enough. None of this would be possible without your eternal support in raising our children. Fareedah, my baby girl. It has and continues to be a pleasure to be

your mum and see you grow into an assertive, confident and intel-
ligent young woman.

To all my siblings, Daniel, Margaret, Osei, Shelia, Cynthia,
Ronnie, Jemima, Charles and Gemma. I'm grateful for all of your
characters, the ups, the downs and the bond that makes us intrin-
sically one.

Big thank you to the team, Kacey, Belinda, Genevive, Irene and
all the others who have played an integral part in making Hair
Lounge the premier Afro hair salon in the UK. Thank you for
being a soundboard to all my crazy ideas and nothing but professional in your approach to work – lots of love.

My editors Emily Robertson and Marianne Tatepo, thank you
for your patience and ability to keep on pushing me for ideas –
we've done something great here.

And last but by no means least, where would I be without my
clients? You guys have been my source of inspiration over the
years, from the interesting conversations to the unique energy
you all bring. You guys literally provide the battery that keeps me
going every morning. This is for you!

I love you all, I always will, and I am grateful.

Charlotte Mensah

ENDNOTES

1. From Motherland to Mother Country

1. http://maa.cam.ac.uk/origins-of-the-afro-comb-6000-years-of-culture-politics-and-identity/
2. Emma Dabiri, *Don't Touch My Hair*, Allen Lane, 2019, p. 38.
3. Sylvia Ardyn Boone, *Radiance from the Waters: Ideals of Feminine Beauty in Mende Art*, Yale University Press, 1986, p. 186.
4. According to Angela Fisher, explorer and photographer. See her book *Africa Adorned*, William Collins, 1984, p. 189.
5. Boone, *Radiance from the Waters*, p. 186.
6. Ayana D. Byrd and Lori L. Tharps, *Hair Story: Untangling the Roots of Black Hair in America*, St Martin's Press, 2001, pp. 6–7.
7. Byrd and Tharps, *Hair Story*, p. 54.
8. Geraldine Biddle-Perry and Sarah Cheang (eds), *Hair: Styling, Culture and Fashion*, BERG, 2008, p. 128.
9. Edward Scobie, *Black Britannia: A History of Blacks in Britain*, Johnson Publishing, 1972.
10. https://blogs.lse.ac.uk/lsehistory/2018/10/10/kwame-nkrumah-lse/

11. Charlotte Mensah, 'Natural Fix', *Black Hair* magazine, October/November 2007.

2. Back to Black

1. Lesley and Phillip Hatton, *Perming and Straightening: A Salon Handbook*, Second Edition, Blackwell Scientific Publications, 1993, pp. 13–15.
2. Hatton, *Perming and Straightening*.
3. Charlotte Mensah, 'Thread Lightly', *Black Beauty & Hair Magazine*, August/September 2009.
4. https://csdt.org/culture/legacy/african/CORNROW_CURVES/culture/african.origins.htm
5. Princess Gabbara, 'Cornrows and Sisterlocks and Their Long History', *Ebony Magazine*, 20 January 2017.
6. Princess Gabbara, 'Everything You Need to Know About Bantu Knots', *Ebony Magazine*, 29 November 2016.

3. Moving On

1. Elaine Woo, 'Comer Cottrell dies at 82; made Jheri Curl available to the masses', *Los Angeles Times*, 8 October 2014.

4. The Apprentice

1. https://www.bbc.co.uk/news/uk-36279845

2. Ayana Byrd and Lori L. Tharp, 'When Black Hair is Against the Rules', *The New York Times*, 30 April 2014.

3. Micha Frazer-Carroll, 'Young Black Brits on Growing up with Hair Discrimination: "It Stays with You"', *Huffington Post*, 5 March 2019.

4. Emma Brazell, 'Risk of cancer increases 45% for black women who dye hair', *Metro*, 10 January 2020.

5. Going into Business

1. Mike Phillips and Trevor Phillips, *Windrush: The Irresistible Rise of Multi-Racial Britain*, HarperCollins, 1998, p. 59.

2. Caryl Phillips, 'The Real Meaning of "Rachmanism"', *The New York Review of Books*, 23 December 2019.

3. Sondra L. Hausner, *Wandering with Sadhus: Ascetics in the Hindu Himalayas*, Indiana University Press, 2007, p. 46.

4. Francesco Mastalia and Alfonse Pagano, *Dreads*, Artisan, 1999, p. 15.

5. Joseph Owens, *Dread the Rastafarians of Jamaica*, Heinemann Educational Books, 1979, p. 18.

6. The Golden Years

1. Lisa Hetfield and Dana M. Britton (eds), *Junctures in Women's Leadership: Business*, Rutgers University Press, 2016, pp. 45–6.

2. Marlène Elias and Judith Carney, 2007, 'African Shea Butter: A Feminized Subsidy from Nature', *AFRICA: Journal of the International African Institute,* 77 (1), 43.

3. https://www.mintel.com/press-centre/beauty-and-personal-care/natural-hair-movement-drives-sales-of-styling-products-in-us-black-haircare-market

INDEX